D1290495

BIRTH

Karen Brody

authorHOUSE®

AuthorHouse™
1663 Liberty Drive, Suite 200
Bloomington, IN 47403
www.authorhouse.com
Phone: 1-800-839-8640

First published by AuthorHouse 7/24/2008

ISBN: 978-1-4343-7741-8 (sc)

Printed in the United States of America
Bloomington, Indiana

This book is printed on acid-free paper.

This play cannot be performed without written consent by the playwright or as part of BOLD (www.boldaction.org).

For my mother, Annette Brody,

and all mothers around the world

In memory of Mary Kroeger

mother, friend, midwife, birth champion

FOREWORD

by Christiane Northrup, MD, FACOG

From the moment I first laid eyes on this play and then had the pleasure of reading it I've thought of this play as *The Vagina Monologues*[1] for birth. This makes perfect sense. After all, the vagina is the birth canal. Or at least it used to be before our culture's preoccupation with technology, scheduling, and fear created the current trend of vaginal bypass surgery (C-section) as the preferred mode of delivery. But I'm getting ahead of myself.

Eve Ensler's Vagina Monologues has helped free vaginas the world over—as well as their owners. Now it's time to do the same for the birth canal—and pregnant women everywhere. And that is the power and glory contained in this magnificent, funny, and wonderfully wise play. And also for BOLD, the organization that is getting the word out about the joys of normal birth.

[1] *The Vagina Monologues* was written by Eve Ensler who also launched V-Day, a nonprofit organization whose mission seeks to end violence against women.

By reading *Birth* and watching it performed women and men everywhere have an instant "ah ha" experience. We are reminded that female bodies know exactly how to give birth normally given the right environment and caregivers. We are reminded that our female bodies were designed by nature for this sublime act of creation. And we are reminded that this short journey down the birth canal to the outside world (known as labor) has profound (and vastly underestimated) benefits for both mother and baby.

I have been a pioneer in the natural birth movement for nearly three decades and have taken a stand for a woman's right to choose a non-medicated, non-medicalized birth for many years. And I have watched in disbelief over the past two decades as thousands of women have colluded with the healthcare profession in having the wisdom of birth buried by technology and fear.

And so it was with great pleasure that I first read *Birth* and then took part in its premiere in New York City on Labor Day 2006 - the birth of the BOLD movement. I felt hope. I felt heartened. How thrilling to see so many women and men of all ages ready and willing to trust their bodies and deepen their connection with the wisdom of birth and the birth canal. How thrilling to hear the real sounds of birth uttered so realistically by the actors. How thrilling to be part of the much-needed change of our current high intervention birth culture and to watch the innate wisdom of the female body in birth so powerfully portrayed on stage.

Kudos to you, Karen Brody, for getting the words and the images just right. And for gifting the world with this moving, life-changing work of art.

Christiane Northrup, MD, FACOG (Fellow of the American College of Obstetricians and Gynecologists) is the author of *Women's Bodies Women's Wisdom* (Bantam 2006) and *Mother Daughter Wisdom* (Bantam 2005).

CONTENTS

INTRODUCTION

Who knew my play would spark a global movement to improve maternity care for mothers? I certainly didn't when I wrote it. In fact, I remember the day I told my husband that after interviewing over one hundred women about their birth experiences I was no longer planning to write a book; I was going to write a play.

"You never wrote a play," he said.

"I'll learn," I replied.

And that's exactly what I did. I asked a neighbor – who wrote grants for a well-respected theater in the Washington, DC area – if he knew a place where playwrights could go to workshop their plays. He directed me to The Playwrights Forum. And the rest, as they say, is history.

I haven't a clue why having two young boys who were three and four-and-a-half didn't stop me. Or how I thought I was going to write a play when my husband traveled a lot for his work. I guess this is what an activist is – a person who commits to something they feel passionate about because they believe it has the power to affect social change. I didn't know it at the time, but that is why I wrote this play. I wanted to swing the birth pendulum to a maternity care system that honors mothers. To put mothers and their birth stories – finally – center stage.

In 2006 after I started BOLD, a global arts-based movement to improve childbirth choices and put mothers at the center of their birth experiences, I quickly found out that I wasn't the only person who thought this mission made sense. My idea resonated with so many other women who had been using traditional methods of educating the public about maternity care, like childbirth education classes and lectures. These women found that even when they dangled an over thirty percent cesarean rate in front of people most weren't getting the urgency of the maternity care crisis and the impact on mothers' lives.

Ironically, except for a small group of academics, most women studies programs today do not educate their students about childbirth and women's rights. After a BOLD performance in Boston in 2007 a women studies professor who had brought students from her class to see the play wondered aloud with the audience, "How come women studies departments don't address this issue?" I'm confused too. And that's why BOLD started our BOLD College Campaign program, so that students - the parents of tomorrow - get information about childbirth early, before they are faced with making important birth choices.

It's not surprising BOLD Organizers have sprouted up all over the world to say childbirth most definitely IS a woman's issue. What I love about BOLD is that instead of doing the typical activist protests with signs and marches BOLD Organizers are producing a play about women's birth experiences as a form of activism, showing audiences what is wrong with the current maternity care system by focusing on what they are for - mother-centered childbirth. Instead of having "My Body Rocks!" carried around as a sign by a pregnant mother at a march audiences all over the world are watching the character Amanda in the play chant "My Body Rocks!"...and they're chanting right along with her. To me, this is the form of BOLD activism maternity care needs today.

There are many themes in this play. Some I intended to write and others just appeared once the pieces of a woman's birth story were complete. I encourage you to read the play aloud and find the themes that resonate for you. If reading the play by yourself doesn't work for you then bring a group of women informally together to read and discuss it. And if you're feeling BOLD, organize a BOLD performance in your neighborhood. It's through people in communities that real, effective change happens.

The moment is now to be BOLD.

Karen Brody
Summer 2008

BIRTH

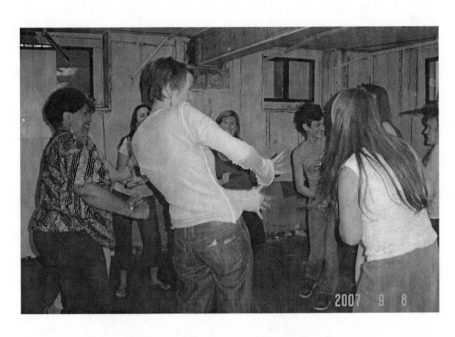

Flagstaff, Arizona cast warming up, BOLD 2007

Cast

AMANDA is a 28-year-old stay-at-home mother of two who lives in the suburbs of Seattle, Washington. She's athletic, mainstream, but liberal and very confident. Her voice is strong and powerful.

BETH is a 35-year-old successful, high-powered computer systems manager from New Jersey. She's friendly, confident and very straight forward.

JANET is a 41-year-old lesbian who is a cameraman for documentary films. She lives in San Francisco. She's happy and very easy-going.

JILLIAN is a 45-year-old stay-at-home mother of four originally from Ohio, but lives in South Texas. She is *very* upbeat, light, funny – Jillian always sees the humor in life. She is optimistic and trusting with a naiveté that's charming.

LISA is a 37-year-old African-American who works for an international women's rights organization in Washington, DC. Lisa is angry, sarcastic and deeply sad about her birth experience.

NATALIE is a 30-year-old successful artist who lives in Albuquerque, New Mexico. She is a strikingly beautiful bi-racial woman, smiles A LOT, is not super "earthy-crunchy" but is open to using alternative health like herbs and acupuncture.

SANDY is a 33-year-old freelance editor for an online magazine. She lives in Wisconsin. She is very likeable, with a "girl-next-door" voice.

VANESSA is a 25-year-old Hispanic woman from New York City who runs her own business. She is strong-willed, funny, with a "couldn't care what anybody thinks about me" attitude.

OTHER CHARACTERS who speak for a short period of time include obstetricians, nurses, midwives, a doula, husbands, mothers and mother-in-laws.

ACT I

Introduction

ACTOR

We always had animals growing up. Puppies and kittens were born just about every year in our house. Human beings are, you know, we're animals.

When a dog is giving birth you leave the mother alone in a dark, safe place away from noise. Can you imagine making a dog in labor lie on her back to push her puppies out, then sticking those wet puppies under lights and poking them?

When I was little I'd watch a dog in labor all day until she moaned and groaned so loud it sounded like a whale giving birth... a howling chant. Her hips swayed back and forth with smooth rhythm. I loved that moment, when the dog knew she was ready and we knew it and the babies started coming out. The dog looked so beautiful.

ALL ACTORS

You're beautiful!

ACTOR

We told her she was doing such a good job.

ALL ACTORS

You can do it!

ACTOR

Nobody was scared. The dog was in pain, but everyone knew it was going to be alright. One by one the wet puppies appeared and snuggled up to their mother. Some fell asleep. Others sucked on her nipples.

I wanted to touch those puppies so bad, grab one to make sure it was alright, but then I'd remember my mother's words: You never take healthy puppies away from their mother. Never.

A mother needs to feel her babies next to her after they're born. A mother giving birth needs some space. Give her some space... love... touch... words of encouragement. This is her moment.

I wanted that same thing preserved when I gave birth.

AN ACTOR

I wanted what my dog got.

Scene 1

AMANDA

I told every friend I know that "I'm going to back up into the labor and delivery room with a martini in hand when I ask for the epidural." That always got a lot of laughs. It felt good to go down the epidural joke line. I mean, who wouldn't want to be numbed from the waist down when you're pushing a baby out? I told all my co-workers that "I'm going to be really mad if the anesthesiologist doesn't meet me right at the entrance to the hospital. I want the epidural at the door!"

Even Oprah – the "love your body" queen – told her millions of
viewers:

OPRAH

Get the epidural ladies!

AMANDA

That's why I only told a few of my closest friends I was really
trying for a natural birth. Deep in my soul I felt like..MY BODY
ROCKS. I can do this. Mammals do it. Giving birth IS natural. But
of course I was also afraid I couldn't do it....so afraid.

Scene 2

JILLIAN

Okay! Where should I start?!! Why don't I start with what I
thought birth was all about... *before* the baby arrived.

Birth to me was all about the "loud, frantic, rush to the emergency
room"! Have you ever seen that scene in "I Love Lucy" where
Lucy is pregnant and she decides she's in labor so she tells Desi:

LUCY

(*in Lucille Ball's ditzy accent*) It's time!

JILLIAN

I love that scene! Desi starts running around shouting:

DESI

(*Heavy Spanish accent*) It's time? You mean, it's *time*?!

LUCY

Yes, it's time!

JILLIAN

(*Jillian gets hysterical laughing.*) Desi finally manages to get a taxi and then he speeds off to the hospital...forgetting Lucy!

To me, birth was ALL about the craziness.

BETH

My sister had a baby when I was a teenager. A total nightmare. I was, like, who wants to go through that?

LISA

I was a footling breech. The OB slapped me three times - the last slap, he said, was —

OBSTETRICIAN

For coming out breech.

NATALIE

My perceptions of birth came from my mother. She always said

NATALIE'S MOTHER

You were an easy birth, Natalie!

NATALIE

And that's what I believed.

SANDY

When my mother had me she was insistent with the doctors and nurses when she got to the hospital that –

SANDY'S MOTHER

This baby is coming out!

SANDY

But they said no – absolutely not – and as she tells it she ended up looking down and my head was practically out.

VANESSA

Growing up I thought birth was a joke. All that grunting and screaming. I thought: that woman needs to calm down!

AMANDA

I wanted to give birth from the moment I saw my cat giving birth in a dark corner of my room when I was ten. She was purring so loud and we were all in awe. I don't know how long the whole labor took…it didn't matter.

JANET

My perceptions of birth came from those tapes they showed in sex ed class in High School. Sex was totally devoid of love and birth was what bad girls did to punish their mothers.

Scene 3

JILLIAN

Okay! My first birth! I thought I was prepared for my first birth, but when "the time" came my husband and I were completely unprepared, nervous wrecks. We were living in New York, two kids in our twenties. I was from the Midwest and thought I was so sophisticated taking out videos on birth from the local video store. I loved New York – you could rent "Independence Day" and a childbirth video all at the same place! I got out a stack of books from the library and watched my videos.

Our neighbor had just had her baby at a birthcenter and she loved it so I thought I'm gonna be one of those savvy New York women and go to a birth center too! I couldn't wait to give birth.

I loved the birth center. Those midwives were just great! I checked my own urine…pulled my own chart. I liked that MY chart was MY chart!

BETH

The first thing you should know about me is that I'm a type A, career person. I work an 80 hour week. I never thought a lot about giving birth, but I did develop a strange obsession in my mid-twenties with episiotomies after my other sister had a baby. Cutting my vagina to get a baby out? Who wouldn't be alarmed? I read everything I could about episiotomies. I talked to every woman I knew who gave birth and I'd always hear how they had an episiotomy and how horrible it was. By the time I got pregnant in my thirties I found out that western medicine does a lot of inducing and then they often do episiotomies on the women they induce. It's all in the medical research. It's hard to find, but I found it. And I didn't like what I read. There was no way I wanted to be cut. So the first thing my OB wrote in my chart was –

OBSTETRICIAN

Fear of episiotomy.

BETH

Then I read an article that showed women who have vaginal deliveries have a greater chance of developing incontinence later in life. Great. I was going to have a baby vaginally and run the risk of having pee dribbling out of me when I got older. No way. The second thing my OB wrote on my chart was –

OBSTETRICIAN

Fear of incontinence.

BETH

Just about every night before I'd go to bed I'd find another alarming fact about vaginal birth. That's when I started thinking c-section. My husband always thought I'd have a c-section. He wanted me to. Who wants to see the area that you find sexual ripped apart? He wasn't the only one encouraging me. I had several OB friends and they all told me:

OBSTETRICIAN FRIENDS

Get the planned c-section, Beth!

BETH

That made me think. If they were staying away from vaginal maybe I should too.

Of course midwives know all about natural birth. But I didn't want a midwife. I wasn't going to deliver in the *bath* water! I find

13

homebirth kind of gross. My cousin gave birth accidentally at home and my friend said she read about a woman giving birth in an elevator and someone bit off the umbilical cord. Yuck! Disgusting. I like the idea of birth being clean.

I told my OB that I don't want any surprises. So the third thing my OB wrote in my chart was:

OBSTETRICIAN

Good candidate for planned c-section.

BETH

Planned? That sounded great!

You know, I'm usually the ultra-natural woman. I buy organic. I did prenatal yoga for all 9 months. But with birth I thought, okay, maybe I don't have to be SO ultra-natural. In the end I chose to have a c-section not because I was afraid to see blood or the pain in labor... and not because of my cleanliness issue. If I had to rate my reasons for choosing a c-section they'd be: 1. The episiotomy thing, 2. Incontinence. I was petrified of incontinence. And 3. Time of year. "Time of year" because I was due January 6th and I was afraid there could be a snowstorm and we wouldn't get to the hospital on time. (*beat*) Nobody's biting off my umbilical cord!

I told everyone I knew about my planned c-section…and everyone thought I was fucking nuts.

AMANDA

The hospital birth class I took? It was a bit of a joke and scared a lot of women. The instructor kept showing us pictures of women giving birth and she'd say –

CHILDBIRTH INSTRUCTOR

Now doesn't this look scary!

AMANDA

I mean, come on. That's not the best thing to say to a room full of pregnant women! I remember telling one woman who was very upset after class one night that as a woman… *You* Rock. *You* Rock! Don't let anybody make you think otherwise.

VANESSA

Women always say, "you'll forget the pain." Trust me, even with an epidural, you don't forget about the pain of a baby coming out of you. How could I forget a sensation that felt like the baby was coming out of my butt? Nobody tells women this. Believe me, you never forget a baby coming out of your butt. I always thought, "how could a baby possibly come out of my vagina?" but when I gave birth - even though I know that's where it came out of - it sure didn't feel like it! Now I tell every pregnant friend the truth: that she's going to swear the baby's coming out the other end – your butt (*beat*). Yes, your butt!

Describe the sensation? Listen, when a baby is coming out of your butt you're going to know it! It's like the worst bowel movement you can imagine. It's like a steam engine coming out of your butt... burning...powerful –

An ACTOR

(*quickly cuts her off*) And your pregnancy?

VANESSA

Terrific! I was all belly. I commuted 2 hours into work every day until the last 6 weeks when I got put on full bed rest because they thought my placenta may be maturing. I had to lie in bed with my feet up for the last month. For someone like me that was death. I'm social. I liked my job. I felt great. I thought, you've got to be kidding me I'm going to lay in bed all day? I hated every minute of it. But I did it. I would do *anything* for my baby.

My husband and I did take a childbirth class. There were ten people in the class.

CHILDBIRTH INSTRUCTOR

How many of you plan on going natural?

VANESSA

Everyone's hand went up except mine. I didn't feel embarrassed. I've always known I would have an epidural. Why would I put myself through pain if there's a way to feel more comfortable? That makes no sense to me. I think everyone has the right to do their own thing, but I'm not a "pain" girl.

CHILDBIRTH INSTRUCTOR

Who in this class does not plan to breastfeed?

VANESSA

Me and two other hands went up. Between my answer to her

first question and then my answer to her second I knew what the instructor was thinking: here's a loser. But I didn't care.

CHILDBIRTH INSTRUCTOR

I'm going to talk about some things in this class that you won't need.

VANESSA

Don't worry, I'll tune you out.

JANET

I never wanted to have a baby. Never played with dolls. I wasn't focused on that. I was a feminist. Volunteered for Planned Parenthood. Definitely anti-establishment. And then the "Lesbian Biological Clock" hit. I wanted to get pregnant in a big, physical way. I was approaching forty and my body said it's time to have a baby. I'd been with my partner, Deb, for seven years. She didn't have this same urge, but after a long conversation on a car trip to the Sierra Mountains three years ago she agreed to it. A year later I was pregnant.

Okay, here's where you're going to think I'm crazy. I know you are. Even though my girlfriend and I had done the whole feminist health thing, we had two midwives as friends, and we did not believe doctors treated women with respect. I actually wanted a medical experience for the birth of our baby. Honestly, I didn't understand how the baby could survive birth. It scared me. How is a baby going to get out of such a narrow space?

I wanted to be within reach of a c-section and an epidural. I know a lot of our friends were let down by my choice, but that's just who I am. I wanted the epidural.

LISA

I suspected I was pregnant the day after I conceived. After a night of passion with Justin I know for sure that is when I got pregnant. I took a pregnancy test a week later and I was right.

I continued to go to the OB/GYN practice that I'd been going to for seven years and at first I generally felt very comfortable with them. But I had never been pregnant before. Now it was different. There were a couple of things that turned me off. First, there was something that bothered me about one of the obstetricians. He would walk in each time for my prenatals and when he saw me he'd say –

LISA'S DOCTOR

Lisa, you're so pregnant!

LISA

Maybe he was trying to sound cheery, but to me it sounded like "Uh-oh, you've crossed the line and now you're one of those. You're no longer young, thin Lisa."

At six months pregnant I spoke to a woman I had worked with for years who had a nine-month-old baby with these doctors.

CO-WORKER

When I was having intense contractions the doctors came in cracking rude jokes with each other about some girl they'd both dated that weekend.

LISA

It got so bad her husband confronted the doctors in the labor room.

HUSBAND OF CO-WORKER

(*angry*) What's up with you?! Is someone gonna pay attention to my wife over here?!!!

LISA

She was thirty-eight and they told her she was this big, big risk. I knew she didn't want to think about it, to deal with the fact that perhaps she didn't actually need the section. I could hear the apprehension in her voice when she told me the outcome.

CO-WORKER

I guess I really needed a c-section. I just need to be happy that I had a healthy baby.

LISA

Okay, I get the healthy baby part...but what about HER?

SANDY

My birth plan was "Whatever-they-wanted." My doctor told me to take the hospital childbirth class. So I took it. At the class the instructor taught us how to breathe with the contractions and then showed this kooky film called "Birth in the Squatting Position."

AN ACTOR(*in the classroom*)

Birth in the *squatting* position?!

SANDY

Yeah, "Birth in the Squatting Position!" The film showed these rural women in some poor country giving birth naturally... squatting, of course. We laughed as we watched it. I didn't connect that a woman like me in the modern world could have my baby like this. Women in cities need to be hooked up to fetal heart monitors for the mother's protection and her baby's! But giving birth in the squatting position? What if the baby lands on its head?!

At 6 months pregnant I started disliking my OB.

OBSTETRICIAN

Your insurance is so bad I'm not even being paid for this. I'm doing this for nothing.

SANDY

Gee, thanks. That made me feel great. He had lots of experience. Lots of *book* knowledge. But he obviously never took a course on compassion in med school. For 6 months my OB had me come in every month until at 7 months my husband's company changed insurance providers – to much better insurance – and then he had me come in every week to see him. I told him I didn't think I needed to go every week. I was the picture of health.

OBSTETRICIAN

(*Obnoxious*) What part of this conversation don't you understand?

GIRLFRIEND

What part of this conversation don't you understand?!!

SANDY

That's right.

GIRLFRIEND

Please tell me you left him.

SANDY

No – I stayed.

GIRLFRIEND

(*gasps*) Why?

SANDY

I thought the birth was only one day. How bad can it be to be
around someone you don't like for one day?

LISA

At 30 weeks pregnant I made the decision to leave my OBs and
have my baby with midwives at a birth center. Midwives seemed
like the perfect fit for me. I picked the most liberal, earth-motherly
midwives I could find... that would take my insurance. The birth
center was located about 30 minutes from my home and job. I
wanted a birth center as opposed to a hospital because I hated
hospitals. Most of them don't smell very good and don't seem
clean. Having a baby isn't a sickness so why do I need to give birth
around sick people?

I LOVED the midwives. At our orientation three granola, earth
mother-looking midwives trotted out in their purple crinkled cotton
tops and Birkenstocks. They showed us a video about giving birth

naturally, gave me some films and books to take out and showed us the birthing rooms. Beautiful wide birthing tubs, mahogany wood everywhere, pretty pictures on the wall. Everything LOOKED great.

NATALIE

(*BIG smile*) At my first prenatal check-up I told my doctor that my mother delivered me in 4 hours.

OBSTETRICIAN

Well, you can forget about that. You'll be a good 18 hours.

NATALIE

Of course this wasn't what I wanted to hear, but I still had hope that my birth would be full of joy. My husband and I took a childbirth class with an amazing instructor.

CHILDBIRTH INSTRUCTOR

Your body was born knowing how to give birth to a baby.

NATALIE

These words inspired and lived in me every day of my pregnancy. I got so into my body when I was pregnant – and just loved thinking about the fact that I was made to do this! I decided to invite a lot of my family members to my birth because I wanted them to know that women were made to give birth. That birth isn't ugly or a condition where something was wrong with me.

I spent most of my pregnancy in this intoxicated state of birthing bliss - reading books like *Birthing From Within* and *The Birth*

Partner - only really coming out of my blissful state when I'd walk into my prenatals.

OBSTETRICIAN

(*looking at chart, not Natalie*) All your tests seem to be in order.

NATALIE

Can I see my tests?

OBSTETRICIAN

(*still looking at chart*) See your tests?

NATALIE

Yes, I'd like to see my test results.

OBSTETRICIAN

(*still looking at chart*) Oh, that's not necessary.

NATALIE

(*to the audience*) "That's not necessary." (*Beat*)You know, sometimes when you're in the middle of something you just don't see what's in front of you…

Scene 4

JILLIAN

Okay! What was my favorite moment of the birth? (*starts to giggle*) I guess I'd have to say – when the baby was born!

VANESSA

When I saw the baby.

AMANDA

The power of seeing my baby.

LISA

(*angry*) I have to say the baby, right?

JANET

Seeing the baby through my legs.

NATALIE

(*BIG smile*) Touching my baby's hair when she was coming out.

SANDY

When they told me I had a healthy baby.

BETH

Absolutely, 100 percent, the second they showed me my baby.

Scene 5

JILLIAN

(*note: Jillian is loud, hysterical and out-of-control in this scene…
really over-the-top drama…like the way birth is typically depicted
in a the movies and on television*).

24

Okay, here's the juicy bit! You may not want to hear this. It's the moment every woman knows is coming, dreads, loves, fears... Birth!!!

My water broke around 2 in the afternoon on a Wednesday. My heartbeat started racing and I said to myself, "This is it, Jillian, get the bags!" I called my husband.

(*to her husband*)
Meet me at the birth center – NOW!

(*to the audience*)
I took a cab. I remember the cab driver was this nice guy from Istanbul. Bright. I think he had his PhD.

TAXI DRIVER
(*said proudly, with heavy Turkish accent*) My wife gave birth to our five children in Turkey. She was knocked out for each one!

JILLIAN
I remember thinking, that's not going to be me – that's something people in small foreign countries like Turkey do. I'm in America!

(*to taxi driver...Jillian's breathing fast and deep*) *That* will never happen to me here! I'm giving birth with midwives at a birth center!

TAXI DRIVER
In my country midwives are what rural women who have no money use.

JILLIAN

(*still breathing fast and deep*) Oh no…midwives are wonderful!
Much, much safer than -

TAXI DRIVER

Here we are. Good luck!

JILLIAN

Thanks!

(*to the audience*)
I walked into the birth center.

(*in her birth*)
(*panicky voice…still breathing heavily*) Hello! Hello! I'm having a
baby!

NURSE

How long have you been in labor?

JILLIAN

(*looks at her watch*) Oh, I don't know, about 20 minutes!

NURSE

(*amused*) Let's have the midwife check you.

JILLIAN

Great!

MIDWIFE

Jillian, you're only one centimeter dilated. Go home and get some sleep.

JILLIAN

Home? Sleep? But my water broke…my bags are packed!

JILLIAN'S HUSBAND

(*panicked*) Where is she?! Where's my wife?!!!!

JILLIAN

Ramone, Honey, I'm in here!

JILLIAN'S HUSBAND

Did you have the baby?!!!!

JILLIAN

No, Honey. I'm in EARLY labor. They think we should go home.

JILLIAN'S HUSBAND

Go home?!

JILLIAN

(*to the audience*)
We felt pretty down after that. I stopped the whole panting routine. My husband held my bag and we jumped in a cab and went back to our apartment. No contractions. Not one tightening sensation in my whole body. It felt like I'd already failed.

But I'm not someone who ever feels sorry for myself! I'd read castor oil can speed up labor so that night before going to bed I drank a large glass of castor oil. Two hours later I started having poop-cramps.

(*bends over like she's having a cramp*)
Ooooh! Cramps… and poop. Cramps… and poop. You get the picture? By eleven in the evening we were back at the birth center and this time I was in full labor. This time the panting was for real.

(*Jillian is now acting out her labor. Labor pains are intense, deeper than before and she's quite hysterical, screaming-her-head off.*)
Oh my God, that hurt like hell! Ooooooh – Eeeeeeh — Aaaaaah!!!!!!! Stop this pain! Stop this pain now!!!

Where's the midwife? Check me! Can somebody check me?!

Three centimeters? Oh no, no, NO!!!! Don't touch me! Nobody touch me!

Aaaaah…here's another one…aaaaaaah! Oooooh! No! No! No!

(*to the audience*) FIVE HOURS LATER.

No more… No more! No more! Check me! Check me! Check me! This can't be happening! I can't do it! I can't do it! Ramone, I can't do this! Okay, okay here's another. Noooooooooo! Aaaaaaaaah! No! No! No! No!

Check me! Check me! Check me now! What? Three centimeters!

Take me to the hospital! Take me there NOW!

(*to audience*) The pain was overwhelming. Mind-blowing pain.

I was exhausted and dehydrated. Really, at that point, I wanted a hospital.

(birthing)
(sarcastic) Hello! Is someone going to give me an epidural? I need it now!

(fast, deep breathing) You're the anesthesiologist? Good. I need an epidural right now. If you're not going to give it to me then just kill me, take the baby and give him to Ramone!

Don't worry, I won't move when the needle goes in. *(her voices gets very low)* I.. need…this. Aaaaaaahh…. Thank you…thank you.

(to audience) I must have thanked the anesthesiologist a million times that morning. He was like my knight-in-shining-armor. That epidural took me out of a very dark, lonely place. Two hours later I delivered my son lying on my back in bed, fully numbed from my waist down. I felt nothing. Nothing. I'm surprised I was able to push him out. It doesn't make a lot of sense.

After birth number one I wanted the epidural, the drugs…the whole package!

Scene 6

BETH

I know women spend their pregnancies trying *not* to have a c-section and here I was planning one, but it made a lot of sense to me. I made the decision to do a c-section eight weeks into my pregnancy – at my second visit. My OB's stats on episiotomies and c-sections were high. So I thought to myself if this guy has such high stats why would I even attempt a vaginal delivery?

My OB never talked me out of it. I figured if my doctor wasn't saying no then, alright, this made some sense.

OBSTETRICIAN

I believe in the right for a woman to choose how she wants to have a baby.

BETH

We were definitely on the same page.

I can't say my OB was this warm and fuzzy guy. He wasn't going to ask how I felt about being pregnant or anything like that. He was a very numbers/science person. My prenatal visits were factual. They lasted about 10 minutes. I got on the scale, peed in a cup, and then saw the doctor for a few minutes. He didn't even know my name or my husband's name for the first 4 or 5 visits. I didn't care. I only cared that he was a good surgeon. My husband felt a little different.

BETH'S HUSBAND

It would have been nice to have him remember our name.

BETH

I can understand that, but we really weren't paying him to remember our name. We were paying him to deliver a healthy baby.

Scene 7

SANDY

Maybe I should have left my OB because I didn't like him. I just kept thinking the way I was being treated is normal. Everything will be okay...the birth is only one day in my life.

I got an ultrasound the day before I went into labor.

OBSTETRICIAN

This is going to be a big baby! Definitely an 8-pounder.

SANDY

That kinda scared me, but again I thought the birth is ONLY one day.

I went to bed early that night and then at 3am my water broke. Wild contractions started immediately. It felt like they were coming from my back and wrapping around my lower body... it was like I was hit by a truck and seeing stars.

(birthing)
Ralph, call the car service!

(to audience) But instead he called his mother.

AN ACTOR

His mother?!

SANDY

That's right. I was, "ooohing and aaaahing," saying "I'm ready!
Let's go!" and he thought his mother would know better than me if
we should go to the hospital. Luckily she's a smart woman.

SANDY'S MOTHER-IN-LAW

Take your wife to the hospital! Now!

SANDY

We arrived at the hospital 30 minutes later and I started throwing
up. Somebody changed me into a hospital gown. I was out of it.
The nurse checked me and she said I was 4 centimeters.

NURSE

(*friendly*) Ready for your epidural?

SANDY

I never thought to say no to the epidural. Every woman I know gets
an epidural. After I got it I had some sensation in my body, but not
much. I slept for 5 hours, but it still took another 18 hours to get
to ten centimeters. I wasn't allowed to eat or drink. They gave me
Pitocin to speed up my labor, and fluids from an IV. But, really, I
just laid there waiting to push.

(*Sandy is now acting out her birth. The atmosphere begins calm
and quiet. Since Sandy has had an epidural she does not feel
tremendous pain so she isn't screaming uncontrollably, but she's
exhausted and she does make loud, intense noises when she's asked
to push.*)

OBSTETRICIAN

(*obnoxious*) This is what I want you to do. Open your legs. (*pauses*). No, wider...no, wider. You can do better than that.

SANDY

It hurts.

OBSTETRICIAN

It doesn't hurt. You've had an epidural. This is a big baby, you're going to have to open your legs as wide as possible or the baby can't get out. Come on...open wider.

SANDY

I'll try...

OBSTETRICIAN

You're going to have to do better than try.

SANDY

(*to audience, sarcastic*) *I'm going to have to do better than try*? Who did he think he was?

OBSTETRICIAN

Now lean back.

SANDY

Lean back? I WANT TO STAND!

OBSTETRICIAN

You can't stand. You had an epidural.

SANDY

If I had only trusted my body, if I had some clue that I didn't have to follow all the rules...that the rules were to protect *him* and his hospital, not me. I know I had an epidural, that I couldn't literally stand, but my body was telling me to stand, not to open my legs up like stretched out scissors. He made me feel like that was the rule. I had to open my legs as wide as possible whether I liked it or not.

I pushed for an hour – propped up a little, but basically flat-on-my-back. The monitors told my OB and the nurses when to tell me to push.

(Sandy acting out birth. NOTE: many of these sounds overlap)

OBSTETRICIAN

(loud and angry) Push!

TWO NURSES

(very serious) ... two, three, four, five, six, seven, eight, nine...

OBSTETRICIAN

(said very quickly as the nurses are counting to ten) Push-push-push-push-push!

SANDY

(overlaps the counting) Grrrrrr...ah!

34

TWO NURSES

Ten!

OBSTETRICIAN and NURSES

(*simultaneously*) Don't push!

(*confused look on Sandy's face*)

Push!!!

Don't push!!!!

Push!!!!

Breathe…

SANDY

(*to audience*) Push, don't push, breathe...I was like, what?! What do I do?! I had no one to focus on...everyone was telling me so many things. I was getting get mad.

(*birthing*)

SANDY

(*breathing heavily*) Could I die?!

OBSTETRICIAN

Of course not. This never happens in the United States.

OBSTETRICIAN and NURSE

(*together*) Push!!!

NURSE

(*Quickly*) One, two, three, four, five, six, seven, eight, nine, ten!

OBSTETRICIAN and NURSE

Don't push!!!

Push!!!

Don't push!!!

SANDY

(*to audience)* Oh, here's the words every mother dreads -

OBSTETRICIAN

(*serious, stern tone*) The baby's heartbeat is dropping.

SANDY

Her heartbeat is dropping?

OBSTETRICIAN

We have to do a c-section.

NURSE

I'll prep for a section.

SANDY

C-section? No...no...I want to push! My BODY wants to push! I'm
in a groove!

OBSTETRICIAN

You can't push. This baby could be 11 pounds! You can't push an
11 pound baby out!

SANDY

*(to audience, angry, sarcastic)*That's funny, he had just told me
the day before that the baby was 8 pounds. How did the baby
gain 3 pounds in less than 24 hours? And...and.. what exactly was
my baby's heartbeat anyway? I don't know. I never asked for a
number! There weren't any loud beeping noises on the monitor and
it definitely wasn't an emergency because I was laying on a gurney
for over 30 minutes in a hallway waiting for them to wheel me into
the OR for the section.

(birthing)
(legs closed, she is breathing to keep the baby in) Aaaah, Aaaah,
Aaaaah, Aaaaah, Aaaaah...

NURSE

Don't push...Don't push.

SANDY

(weeping) I just...I just want to push her out!!

NURSE

Don't push!

SANDY

(to audience) I was using all the stupid breathing techniques for pushing that I'd learned in the hospital childbirth class, but instead I was using them to like hold her in. And then after I spent 30 minutes holding her in during the section the anesthesiologist said to me right after my baby was born:

ANAESTHESIOLOGIST

Don't cry.

SANDY

How can I *not* cry? My baby was just born?!

ANAESTHESIOLOGIST

It's important not to cry because you could choke.

SANDY

I could choke...well..Excuse me for crying at the birth of my first child!

(to audience) After they pulled my baby out she scored a 9 on her apgar. A nine out of ten on the test that indicates how healthy she is. She scored a 9 and an hour before she was born she was going to die? I just don't buy it. Here's another thing I don't buy: the baby's weight. My 11 pound baby weighed in at 6 pounds 6 ounces. I trusted my doctor...I figured he knew better than me.

You know, the only good thing about the day I had my c-section was that my mother was there after the birth when I got to my room. She hadn't planned to come down – it was a long drive – but she said the minute Mitch told her I was in labor she got in the car and started driving.

SANDY'S MOTHER

Sandy, I'm here Honey. It's gonna be okay.

SANDY

Mommy...mommy...I need you.. please hold me…

(to audience) I wasn't comfortable after the section, but everything seemed normal. Two days later in the hospital I started to feel like something was going wrong. I was throwing up, unable to eat. It was pretty bad – projectile vomiting.

(to nurses)
Could someone PLEASE help me?! Nurse? I need a nurse! Help me!

(to audience) For 45 minutes I kept trying to get a nurse to come in and help – I kept ringing the nurses' bell. Finally, a friend walked in and I asked him to get the nurse.

NURSE

What's the problem?

SANDY

What's the problem? I've been sitting in my vomit almost an hour and my stomach muscles have just been sliced making it impossible for me to get out of bed. Do I need a better problem?! I felt like a bad patient. I finally wasn't following all the rules! I screamed at the nurse: YOU'RE IN THE HAPPIEST PLACE IN THE HOSPITAL! THE MATERNITY WARD! WHY ARE YOU NOT HAPPY?! They treated me like how dare I ring their bell! Meanwhile, after a congo-line of doctors paraded through my room to figure out why I was throwing up and running a fever, they found out I had a paralyzed bowel brought on by the c-section. I was in the hospital for 10 days. Even after leaving the hospital my body didn't feel normal for over a year. But... birth is "just one day," right?

Scene 8

JILLIAN

Okay! Birth number two!

I was now in total agreement with that taxi driver from Istanbul that the best way for a modern woman to have a baby was to be completely knocked out. I thought, he was right, natural birth was something rural women who had no money did. I was paying for "the works" this time from the beginning. Get this – I was so obsessed with them having my epidural ready that I met with the anesthesiologist before the birth so he could see my back!

I wanted the quickest, fastest epidural known to mankind. My feeling was: do ANYTHING to get the baby out.

I'd like to think of my epidural as an "Empowering Epidural." I got into the hospital, suffered for 3 hours until I was dilated to 4 centimeters and then "wham-bam" thank you, Mr. Anesthesiologist... my epidural! (pauses, then takes a deep breath).

Aaaahh...Empowering epidural! Sometimes a woman just needs an epidural.

I didn't personally think an epidural was the "right" thing to do, I knew I could get a horrible spinal headache for days or weeks afterward, but I didn't want to repeat the circus at my first birth.

This birth was pretty straight forward. Twelve hours. Lots of beeping machines, nurses coming in and out, my husband waiting for me to dilate to 10 so I could push. Then the nurse and doctor screamed:

NURSE AND DOCTOR

Push!!!!!!!!!!!!!!

JILLIAN

And the nurse started counting

NURSE

One, two, three, four…

JILLIAN

I felt totally disconnected. But that didn't matter. The goal of this birth was clear in my mind: to get the baby out of me healthy…not to have a euphoric experience for me and the baby. Get the baby out and don't die in the process. That's what the epidural did for me.

Scene 9

LISA

A few weeks after I had switched from obstetricians to midwives, at my 33 week checkup, the midwives told me –

MIDWIFE ONE

The baby's head is down.

LISA

(*Looks pissed off*) The baby's head is down? I'd swear on a stack of bibles my baby's head wasn't down. I could feel the weight of his head tucked under my rib cage. His head wasn't down. At every visit after that I kept telling them I think my baby's head is up like a breech baby, not down.

MIDWIFE TWO

No, there's a foot in your rib cage. The baby's head is down.

LISA

A week after my due date, at 41 weeks, one of the midwives told me if I didn't give birth that weekend they'd send me to get an ultrasound. By Monday I was still not in labor so off I went for the ultrasound. Remember, I knew exactly when I'd conceived. In my mind I wasn't 41 weeks pregnant I was 39. In MY mind, this baby wasn't late. But I was happy to be getting an ultrasound. Now we'd finally know the position of the baby.

AN ACTOR

Up or down?

42

LISA

Surprise, surprise the ultrasound showed my baby's HEAD in my rib cage. He was breech.

Scene 10

AMANDA

My pregnancy and birth mantra was, *My Body Rocks!* Maybe it wasn't realistic to so profoundly believe "My Body Rocks," but I grew up with strong female role models. In fact, this notion that men control situations or have an upper hand is not in my reality. It really floors me when people think that way. Being a woman means doing whatever you want to do. Being strong. So when I went into labor whenever my uterus felt like two cymbals had just smashed up against its sides during a contraction and I couldn't see the finish line I'd think: My body rocks…My BODY rocks!

Who was at the birth? My husband. Oh – and a doula. Definitely a doula.

ALL ACTORS

A what?

AMANDA

It's funny, a lot of people say, "A what?" It's incredible how few people know about doulas. A doula's like your mom, your best friend and your childbirth educator rolled into one. She's there with you, throughout the labor. She's clued in that birth is woman's work and that many women want other women to support them when they're having a baby. Not replace the husband or anything like that. Just be there – for me. Woman to woman. I'd have been a nervous wreck without Jamie, my doula. It's like, my husband and I went into the hospital and all we had was Plan A – have the baby naturally. We didn't have a "Plan B." We didn't plan for the moment I discovered that my one remedy for pain – massage – was exactly what I hated the most. My doula had alternatives – a birthing ball, visualizations. Having a doula meant my husband didn't have to know everything. He could relax. We could *all* relax.

[*Birthing. Her birth sounds are intense and loud, but she is not hysterical.*]
I'll know when it's time, Dave. *I'm* the woman. I'll know when to go to the hospital. The contractions are like heavy tickles. It's *not* time.

Aaaaaaaah.. .Aaaaaaaaah. . .Aaaaaaaaaaah. I'm going for a walk!

(*to audience*)
I did power walking for an hour. I called it my I AM WOMAN HEAR ME ROAR walk. When I got back home I still didn't think it was time to go to the hospital.

(*birthing*)
Aaaaah...yes! Aaaaah...yes! [*a little more anxious*]…Aaaaah... yes! Let's call the doula! Jamie, it's not time, right? It's not time? (*breathing heavily*)What, it's time? It's time?!

[*to audience*]
I'm not often wrong, but I was then. It was time to go to the hospital.. .*definitely* time. I think in the back of my mind I kept

thinking "Not now" because I was afraid of being one of those out of control mothers who asks the nurses to check her and she's only 1 centimeter dilated. Also, I thought I'd know when I was in heavy labor. How could a woman not know?

It was only when I got in the car with Dave and Jamie that it was clear to me I was in labor.

(birthing)
Here's another one...here's another one...here's... hold my hand, Jamie! Aaaaaaaaaaaaaah...Aaaaaaaaaaaaah...Aaaaaaaaaaaaah..... My body ROCKS!...My body ROCKS!

DOULA

Your body *rocks,* Amanda!

[*to audience*]

AMANDA

When we got to the hospital I was 6 centimeters. I was sure the baby would be out in the next 30 minutes. But, no, wrong again. My labor slowed down. My body went into what I can only describe as "protective cat mode." If my body could speak it would have said:

An ACTOR
NOBODY'S COMING NEAR ME!

AMANDA

Here's where my doula was crucial, she said to me:

45

DOULA

Feel your strength, Amanda. Imagine all the women who have birthed before you, holding hands, cheering you on, smiling at you and your baby. They know you can do it. Feel their strength...feel YOUR strength.

AMANDA

(*lots of birth sounds*) Aaaaaaaaaaaaah...Aaaaaaaaaaaaaah... Aaaaaaaaaaaaaah...My body rocks! My body rocks...

DOULA

Your body ...

(*to audience*)

AMANDA

Rocks. This was a pretty important image for me to hold onto when I gave birth. Imagery worked like magic. When Jamie would tell me "My body rocks" I imagined myself standing on the top of a mountain showing off my beefy muscles. That woman on top of the mountain could give birth. She ROCKED!

We walked the hallways for an hour. Me, Dave and Jamie. I knew how much Dave wanted to touch me. We had an agreement that he was going to give me a kick-ass massage during labor. I thought that's what I wanted. But what I really wanted was to be alone, inside myself, with the encouraging voice of a woman in the background, telling me I was strong. That my body *rocked.*
Two hours after I'd entered the hospital I had stripped down to just a little tank shirt and I was ready to push.
(*birthing*)

My body's pushing! Is that okay?! Where's the doctor?

NURSE

He'll be here in two minutes.

AMANDA

I can't wait two minutes to push...I'm pushing now!

TWO NURSES

[*loud*] One, two, three, four...

AMANDA

I don't want to do the counting! Didn't you read my birth plan?

TWO NURSES

Five, six…

AMANDA

Just let ME push!

TWO NURSES

Seven, eight, nine…

AMANDA

Let me push!
[*starts chant-like labor sounds*] Aaaaaaaaaaaah. . .Aaaaaaaaaaah..
.Aaaaaaaaaaaah...
[*doctor walks in*] Hello, Dr. Rickie!

[*chanting gets much louder*] Aaaaaaaaaaahh...Aaaaaaaaaah...

Aaaaaaaaaaaah...MY BODY ROCKS! MY BODY ROCKS! MY
BODY ROCKS!

*(The doula gets the audience chanting "My Body Rocks!" She's
enthusiastic - like a cheerleader. The point is to get the audience
really wild and chanting throughout Amanda's entire labor. The rest
of the cast can even go out into the audience and get them chanting.)*

DOULA

Everyone...say it with her! My Body Rocks!

AMANDA

MY BODY ROCKS! MY BODY ROCKS! MY BODY ROCKS!

DOULA

Keep it going!

AMANDA

Aaaaaaaah... Aaaaaaaaaah....Aaaaaaaaaaaah!MY BODY
ROCKS!MY BODY ROCKS! MY BODY ROCKS!

DOULA

Louder! Say it with her!

AMANDA

MY BODY ROCKS! MY BODY ROCKS! MY BODY ROCKS!

(very loud so the audience hears her over their chanting)
Ooooooooooh, ooooooooooh, ooooooooooh! It's burning! It's burning!

DAVE

I see the head!

DR. RICKI

This is it!

AMANDA

MY BODY ROCKS!!!!!MY BODY ROCKS!!!!!!!!!!!!!!!

(Amanda pushes the baby out while the audience keeps chanting and then she waves her hands authoritatively in the air to silence the audience)

Dexter shot out of me like a cannon ball.

End of Act 1

Act 2

Scene 1

JILLIAN

Can a woman really give birth like a dog ? I sure do hope so!

JANET

I don't want to give birth like a dog. That sounds so –

VANESSA

Nasty!

SANDY

Nasty? Imagine how quiet it would be. Nobody making loud noises.

LISA

Everyone listening to you.

BETH

You are ALL wrong. Totally wrong. Research shows that dogs stretch more easily than women do. A woman can't have an easy vaginal birth like a dog.

AMANDA

But that's not the point.

VANESSA

That sounds like the point to me!

NATALIE

A woman's never going to open as easily or wide as a dog. It's about the atmosphere. When the atmosphere is right – and a woman feels safe – I believe she WILL open.

Scene 2

JILLIAN

(to audience, excited, happy) Okay!...birth number three! We were in Texas for that birth. I was working at a Spanish language school as an administrator. So boring – don't even ask. One day this student walks in my office, asks me some questions and after two seconds I'm like, I love this woman. She knows something. We go on and on like women do – blah, blah, blah – and then I find out: she's a midwife. Well, you know what I think about midwives. "No way, don't come near me, pain is out of my equation when it comes to birth. I got the empowering epidural."

My husband and I were thinking about having a third child at the time, but definitely not with a midwife. Still, I was curious.

MIDWIFE

I have one woman due in 4 weeks.

JILLIAN

I don't know why, call me crazy – which my husband always

does – I became very interested in this midwife and in going to this birth. (*smiles, giggles*) No, I think I could honestly say I was obsessed! I was going to this birth!

By the end of our conversation in my office I had asked the midwife if I could attend the birth.

MIDWIFE

No.

JILLIAN

Well she said no, as in not "no." More like a no as in

MIDWIFE

Jillian, if you do your homework, read these 4 books on childbirth, then...maybe.

JILLIAN

Maybe was good enough for me! I ran to the bookstore after work and started reading – books by Ina May Gaskin and Michel Odent (*note pronunciation is French: Mee-shel Ohdont*). I remember something that Ina May said in her book really stuck with me about a pregnant mother's body.

INA MAY

Remember this, for it is as true as true gets: Your body is not a lemon.

JILLIAN

Not a lemon! (*laughs loudly, but wonders*)

Scene 3

VANESSA

I thought it was great to be 2 centimeters dilated and 85 % effaced 2 weeks before my due date. The baby's coming any minute, right?

AN ACTOR

Wrong.

VANESSA

Three and a half weeks later I had progressed - a HALF a centimeter to two and a half centimeters. I was 10 days past my due date.

OBSTETRICIAN

Vanessa, we need to induce you.

VANESSA

I didn't care about being induced. In fact, the night before I got the best sleep of my pregnancy. At 5.30 am we got to the hospital. By 7 they inserted a pill into my cervix.

NURSE (*cheery*)

Here's your pill!

VANESSA

I have no idea what it was just that it was meant to start the contractions. And it did. Those contractions were strong.

Grraaaaaaaaaaaah!

I was pissed. Not pissed at the pain. Just pissed off in general. I looked at my stressed-out husband.

(Birthing)
What do they think I'm gonna do - sit here for hours! Somebody check me!

NURSE

Two and a half centimeters.

VANESSA

You gotta be kidding me!

(to audience) The whole experience was kinda strange. Strong contractions, nobody around. It must have been a busy night in the maternity ward. It didn't really matter to me. I could handle the contractions. I knew I was going to get the epidural, but now I thought to myself: Vanessa, save the pain relief for when it gets really bad. I knew it was going to get worse. It had to.

NURSE

You're three centimeters!

VANESSA

I got another pill in my cervix. Then the contractions REALLY got going. That's when those butt contractions started. Extreme pressure in my butt.

AN ACTOR

In your butt?

VANESSA

In my head that baby was knocking on my butt! My whole body was going up and down like a snake who's being attacked. My husband said-

VANESSA'S HUSBAND

Can you sit still?!

VANESSA

No! I can't sit still. You try to sit still with a *baby* coming out of your butt!

HUSBAND

You're out of control!

VANESSA

I wasn't out of control. If I was so out of control I would have got the epidural! I didn't want the epidural – yet.

NURSE

You're 5 centimeters!

VANESSA

At this point my husband said to me:

HUSBAND

You're nuts! Get the epidural! We all need some rest.

VANESSA

Call me crazy for not getting the epidural then, but I knew I was okay.

NURSE

We need to break your water to speed things up.

VANESSA

I said okay, no problem. But – ay yai yai – the pain got a lot worse
after that.

NURSE

Six centimeter! Ready for your epidural?

VANESSA

(to audience) I still wasn't ready. I just wanted them to dull the
pain. So they gave me this shot – I don't know what it was – all I
know is that 2 minutes after the shot it did not just dull the pain…I
felt like I was knocked unconscious. I got the shakes. My whole
body was not right. It felt like I was heavily sedated. I screamed
for my husband to -

(screaming wildly) Do Something!

(to audience) He was in the room with our family watching a
soccer game. My mother, father, 2 sisters, and his sister, brother,
mother and father. They were all sitting on chairs watching soccer.
A part of me wanted to tell everyone to get out. Get the fuck out
of my birth! But I knew they all wanted to be there when the baby
came out. And a big part of me wanted them there too. They are
family, you know.

My husband did stop watching the game at this point and held my hand. It took about 30 minutes before the medication wore off and then I felt everything. All that butt pain.

(birthing)
GIVE ME THE EPIDURAL!!!!

(to audience) I thought I was going to die.

AN ACTOR

Die?

VANESSA

Yes. Honestly, I don't know how women go natural. You don't get a medal for doing it natural so why do it? I know it's only four more to ten centimeters and then I could start pushing this baby out. But those last four are the worst.

(Vanessa gets her epidural)

Getting an epidural was a great moment, even with the creepy feeling I got when the anesthesiologist stuck that needle in my back. I didn't care how strange it felt for the lower half of my body to go numb.

After the epidural I still felt contractions, but the epidural dulled everything a lot. It was great. Now I could watch the soccer game with everyone else!
I think men should be jealous that women can give birth. Once you take the pain away, it's not so bad. I'm just glad there is pain relief.

Everything went great after the epidural.

NURSE

Your blood pressure is dropping.

VANESSA

Oh, but I always forget about this part.

(*loud beeping noise. Vanessa's eyes nervously look at the doctor and nurses*) What's wrong?!

NURSE

Your blood pressure is dropping and the baby's fetal heart tones are dropping.

VANESSA

Hey! Why is everybody running around?

OB

Get an O-2 tube on her.

VANESSA

What's this tube?

(*an oxygen tube goes over her face preventing her from talking. Bright lights go on*)

OB

(*Talking to the nurse, not Vanessa*) This may be a c-section.

VANESSA

(*she rips the oxygen mask off*) Say what? C-section?! Forget that!
I'm pushing this baby out!

OB

Get the suction!

(*nurse gives doctor vacuum suction*)

VANESSA

I MEAN BUSINESS! Haaaaaaaaaaaaaaaaaaaaaaaaaaaaaaaaaaaaaah!

OB

(*uses suction to get the baby out.*)

NURSE

The baby's out!

VANESSA

Thank God that baby didn't come out of my butt! The baby was fine
when he came out. Totally healthy.

Not me...

NURSE

Forth degree tear.

VANESSA

They were sewing me up for a LONG time after the birth. I just
wanted to close my legs for one freaking minute. I just wanted to
be finished. To be alone with my baby. You know, my body ached

to hold him.

Oh, where was my family? They were all in the room with me. (Beat) Still watching soccer.

Scene 4

BETH

First thing Monday morning is the best time to plan surgery. You want a Monday so you don't have to be in the hospital over the weekend. Everyone says the quality of the nursing staff is worse on weekends. I can't tell you if that's true because my c-section was scheduled for 8am on a Monday.

When we left at 5.30am. I felt great, like this is going to be a piece of cake. I felt so good *I* was videotaping my husband leaving the house!

I have to admit, once we checked in at the hospital I did start to get really nervous. It's typical of me to plan, plan, plan and then not realize what I'm doing. This was major surgery. Everyone told me, but that didn't hit until I was getting prepped.

But I loved my c-section. I can't comprehend why anyone would want to have vaginal pain. All those ice packs during recovery. The only thing I didn't like was that the doctor was late. My 8am surgery started at noon. He wasn't late because he was busy with another patient. He just got the time wrong. He thought the surgery was at noon.

I did think it was weird that the OB hardly paid any attention to me during surgery.

OBSTETRICIAN

(*friendly*) Hi. How ya doing? Lie down.

BETH

During the surgery the OB was actually talking to the nurses about what he did over the weekend. He asked me once how I was feeling. But, like I said, I didn't hire him to be nice. I hired him to deliver a healthy baby.

My husband and I did have one strict rule during the c-section. That he couldn't look horrified when he saw my guts out. I didn't need to be reminded that my guts were hanging out for 30 minutes.

I also insisted my husband tell jokes throughout the section.

(in birth)
Jeff, tell everybody a joke!

BETH'S HUSBAND

Naaa..

BETH

Yes! Yes! Tell a joke!

BETH'S HUSBAND

Alright…alright… How many Obstetricians does it take to screw in a light bulb?

(to audience)

BETH

That's my husband, always joking! I loved it.

(then silence…*back in her birth*)

Ooooh…that was quite a tug!

BETH'S HUSBAND

Uh, doc…everything alright over there?

OBSTETRICIAN

Absolutely! We just have to use some forceps to bring your little guy down so I can get him out.

BETH'S HUSBAND

Okay! You do your thing and I'll do mine! Okay…where were we… did you ever hear the one about the three hunters?

(to audience)

BETH

The whole experience was exactly what I wanted. I didn't have anxiety. I didn't have to deal with all that craziness women go through giving birth. I wanted easy… and I got it.

Of course I'll always be curious about the whole natural childbirth thing. I know there are lots of things in life I will never experience. I'll probably never climb the Himalayas…or Mount Kilimanjaro… but I'll always wonder…

Scene 5

JILLIAN

Remember the midwife who said to me "read these 4 books" and then MAYBE I could attend Abby's homebirth? Well.. (*giggles*)I devoured all 4 books the midwife gave me in one week! I think she was shocked.

(*to the midwife*) So now can I go?

I thought I'd still get a maybe...I didn't even know this midwife – or the woman giving birth... but instead she said

MIDWIFE

I'll check with Abby to see if it's okay.

JILLIAN

I don't know why I felt so excited, but inside of me I thought, "Yes!" When I told my husband he was eating a ham and cheese sandwich on our recliner in our living room when I told him...

JILLIAN'S HUSBAND

(*chokes on sandwich*) Midwives! You hate midwives!

JILLIAN

I don't hate midwives, Ramone. I don't know...there's something about this midwife. She's different.

JILLIAN'S HUSBAND

Different? Different? Okay, that's fine. But what about blood?

JILLIAN

Blood?

JILLIAN'S HUSBAND

You hate blood! You can't watch any of those surgery shows – they always make you squeamish. How are you doing to deal with birth if you can't deal with surgery shows?

JILLIAN

Ramone, there may be a lot of blood. You're right. But giving birth isn't a 911 incident.

(to audience, giggles) That really shut him up!

So I went to the birth. Wow... to watch a baby being born like that. I hadn't seen anything like it before. It was beautiful. Abby made these incredible howling noises. I wouldn't have thought the sound of a whale in distress would be too nice!

ABBY

(slowly) Waaa...hooo!!!!!!!!!! Waaa...hoo!!!!!!!!!!!!

JILLIAN

Abby waahoo-ed for hours. After it was over I walked out thinking: I want what SHE got. I began to seek safe passage. I finally began to walk through all my birth baggage.

Scene 6

NATALIE

(*BIG smile*) It was a beautiful, sunny day when I went into labor. I remember the birds were chirping, the air was so clean. I felt great. I knew I was in labor, my body felt so alive. George and I decided to go for a walk in a nearby park. We stood in the park and danced with the sun beating down on my face. (*starts to belly dance*) I belly danced with each contraction and it felt awesome and right and as things should be. There was no sense in my body that we needed to go to the hospital. Nothing. I wanted to be in that park dancing with George forever.

(*giggling and smiling*)

GEORGE

You look like the happiest woman in the world today.

NATALIE

And I was. My baby was coming and my body was so ready, so full of joy that this day had finally come. George held my hands and we swayed for hours in the park.

About 4 hours later the contractions picked up and I thought should probably call the doctor's office.

NURSE

You're in labor? Go to the hospital immediately.

NATALIE

(*to audience*) I didn't want to go to the hospital. I wasn't ready. I told the nurse this. She wasn't happy with me.

NURSE

At least come to our offices to get checked.

NATALIE

This made sense. So we walked home and slowly got in the car to go see the doctor.

NURSE

You're five centimeters! You have to go to the hospital right now.

NATALIE

My body was telling me not to go. I wasn't ready. But then I decided this was my doctor and I trusted her so I better do what I was told. At the hospital everything felt very serious. Nobody was smiling. My body felt completely different. I didn't even feel any contractions anymore, but I was still smiling, knowing my baby was coming and that I would soon push her out. Five minutes later my family showed up. And five minutes after that the doula I hired walked in with a boom box, electric candles to dim the room and a birthing ball.

DOULA

Natalie, dance with George...

NATALIE and GEORGE

(*dancing with soft music playing...Natalie is trying to get into her*

66

birth, but is more just going through the motions)

NATALIE

Oooooooooooo….aaaaaaaaaaaaaaaaaaaaaaaaaaaaa……
oooooooooooooo…..aaaaaaaaaah…
(gets on the birthing ball)

(to the audience) I was doing ALL the right things. Dancing with George, swaying on the birthing ball, smiling, wanting to show my family that I CAN do this. I so wanted to be an example to them that women CAN give birth without all the craziness.

(She has a fake smile on her face) Ooooooooooo…
aaaaaaaaaaaaaaaaaaaaaaaa…….ooooooooooooooo…….
aaaaaaaaaaaaaaah….

(looks nervously as nurse comes in) Aaaaaaaaaaaaaa…
ooooooooooooooo…..

NURSE

Want an epidural?

NATALIE

No! No!

(to audience) I didn't want the epidural. I wasn't in a lot of pain. But I know my husband really wanted me to get one.

GEORGE

You're tired, Nat.

NATALIE

No! I'm not getting an epidural!

DOULA

Let's try saying these words, Natalie...Ooopen...Ooopen..

NATALIE

(*likes doula's suggestion, starts to smile again*) Yes...yes...
Ooopen! Ooopen! Ooopen!

NATALIE and DOULA

Ooopen...Ooopen...Ooopen...

NATALIE

I went on like this for about another 15 minutes and then my OB
walked in.

OB

Natalie, we need you to dilate faster.

NATALIE

Faster? But I'm fine...I'm fine!

OB

You're only at 6 centimeters and you've been in the hospital 5
hours.

NATALIE

I don't want any drugs!

OB

Okay. We can start with breaking your water.

NATALIE

(*looks at her doula and husband*) Break my water?

DOULA

(*to doctor*) Dr. Barter, can we have a minute?

OB

(*a little annoyed*) Okay.

DOULA

Natalie, what do YOU want? This is YOUR birth.

NATALIE

I want to be alone. I NEED to be alone!

(*to audience*)

So I got to be alone…but I could see the doctor was pissed…and…
and…I felt like a BAD girl… so eventually I said okay…okay…
BREAK MY WATER!

OB

(*breaks her water*) Okay. Done.

NATALIE

(*the contractions get MUCH more painful*) Aaaaaaaaaaaaaaaaaaah!
Aaaaaaaaaaaaah! This is too much!

DOULA

Where does it hurt?

NATALIE

EVERYWHERE! Aaaaaaah…Aaaaaaaaaaaaaaaaah….Aaaaaaaaaaa
aaaaaaaaaaaaaaaaaaaaaah!

NURSE

Epidural now?

NATALIE

I didn't want an epidural! I just didn't want one. But then I looked
over at George and he was so upset…he was crying…and I said

(to nurse) Okay…give me an epidural.

(to audience) After that I got several hours of sleep. I felt so
dejected. I sent my family out of the room. I didn't want them to
see THIS…I didn't want them to think this was what birth was all
about. Everything felt all wrong. About 4 hours after my epidural
the doctor came in.

OB

We're going to need to do a c-section.

NATALIE

A c-section? No! I can push my baby out! Why do I need a c-
section?

OB

We're concerned you're taking so long to dilate.

NATALIE

So long? You have to give me more time! How much more time can I have?

OB

(*checks his watch*) Okay. You have one hour.

NATALIE

(*to audience*) One hour to get to ten? A deadline! I didn't have time to think how crazy this was, I just had to get to ten. My doula encouraged me to close my eyes and get back into that space I was in at the park, imagining the sun beating down on me, the birds chirping, dancing with George (*she and George begin dancing together*)…I dug DEEP inside myself and began to feel my rhythm again, the joy, my connection to my baby…(*she starts to authentically smile*)…and the contractions came back…we could see them on the monitor…they were there…strong…powerful… and like magic in one hour I had made it. (*BIG smile*) I was ten.

OB

You have one hour to push. If the baby isn't out in an hour we're doing a c-section.

NATALIE

More deadlines! I wasn't happy, but I began to get myself mentally ready to push. I thought: I CAN do this! I CAN do this! And then the nurses began counting.

NURSES

(*softly counting to nine*) PUSH! Two, three, four, five, six, seven, eight, nine, ten…

NATALIE

I bared down to push with everything I had in me…but… I could feel nothing. The numbness from the epidural left me without control of anything from my waist down. I tried again and again to push when they yelled

NURSES

PUSH!

NATALIE

But there was no feeling…nothing…I didn't know how to push…it was all overwhelming. At one hour the OB stood up.

OB

Prep for a section.

NATALIE

I looked at George and my doula…my doula started doing the colors…the colors we had practiced that I'd visualize if I was going to have a c-section but I kept thinking:

I DON"T WANT TO DO THE FUCKING COLORS!
I don't want to do this anymore! I knew I could push my baby out. So I told the two nurses in the room that I was going to push again and they said no but I said "Yes!" and when the doctor walked

back in the baby's head was crowning. I put my hand down…and I could feel her hair. (*BIG smile*) My baby was coming! I was so excited…I was going to do it…but just before I went to push her head out I felt something cold on my vagina and…and…

Noooooooooooooooooooooooooooooooooooooooooooooooooooo! Don't cut me!!!!!!

Please don't cut me! Don't cut me! And she cut me… she cut me…

(*LONG pause*)
My vagina will NEVER be the same.

Scene 7

JANET

I know, I know I should have been going to midwives…but my mind told me that a hospital is safer than midwives. The bottom line is I want a healthy baby. My baby's health comes before any kind of earthy-crunchy birth experience. My OBs were the closest thing to a midwife you could get. Warm. Funny. Hip. They could have been your friends. Their practice was busy. They delivered at one of the five premiere baby hospitals. I liked that. I felt I could surrender myself to their expertise.

One week past my due date I was still pregnant. I tried everything to start my labor. Our two midwife friends brought over red raspberry tea to drink and that didn't do anything. I tried squatting a lot, walking…let's see, nipple stimulation, masturbation…I even baked cookies because a friend told us that stirring the batter would bring on contractions! But nothing was making me go into labor.

My doctor wanted to induce. She always induces at 41 weeks. I knew the risks of induction - that one intervention can lead to another - but I felt like induction was going to work for me. So Deb, our friend Tish and I went to the hospital. At 6am they induced me. Four hours later I was in full labor.

(birthing)

JANET

Aaaah...ooooh....aaaahhh...oooohh...Let the pain out!... Let the pain out! ...aaaah....ooooh...aaaah....ooooh... Let the pain out!

JANET

(to audience) The contractions were hard. They couldn't give me the epidural until I was at 3 centimeters so I had to deal with it. After 4 hours I finally got to three. I got the epidural. After that, the pain almost disappeared – it was really incredible. I was sleeping through my labor! That's until –

(Birthing)
(There's a loud beeping sound. She is jolted from her sleep.)
What was that?!! Deb, get the nurse. What's that beeping? I'm feeling a little dizzy. I think I may pass out. Tish?... Deb?

NURSE

Low blood pressure.

JANET

Fine, give me anything... (*dizzy*) Deb?

(*to audience*) They got ephedrine into me just in time and I didn't pass out. It was all a bit scary and I thought, okay, now I understand what they mean about not intervening in a natural process. The epidural caused my blood pressure to drop and then the baby's heart tones dropped and that was why I got dizzy. That was my lesson in medicalized birth. From then on they monitored the baby's heartbeat. Three hours later I was 10 centimeters. They told me to push. Tish was on one side, Deb was on the other, the obstetrician and two labor and delivery nurses were at the end of the bed... and I was in the middle.

(*She has an epidural so is not screaming wildly. The contractions feel intense when she's pushing - like she's constipated and pushing out stool.*)

OBSTETRICIAN

(*loud, with lots of enthusiasm, like a soccer mom*) Come on, Janet, you can do it! Come on, Janet, you can do it!

TWO NURSES

Come on, Janet! Push! Push! Come on, Janet!

DEB and TISH

Push! Push Janet!

JANET

Grrrrrrrrrrr...ah! Is the baby okay? Is the baby okay?!

NURSE ONE

He's fine!

NURSE TWO

Here comes another contraction. Ready…

OBSTETRICIAN and NURSES

Push! … two, three, four, five, six, seven, eight, nine, ten!

JANET

(*pushing hard, but quietly, very inward – not loud*) Grrrrrr....aah!
Grrrrrrr....aah! Is the baby okay? Is the baby okay?

OBSTETRICIAN

Yes! Yes! Come on, Janet, you can do it!

NURSE ONE

You're doing great, Janet!

OBSTETRICIAN and TWO NURSE and DEB and TISH

PUSH! … two, three, four, five, six, seven, eight, nine, ten!

JANET

(*heavy breathing, overlapping counting*) Grrrrrrr...aah! Grrrrrr...
aah!

(*after number counting*) Is the baby okay?

(*everyone is silent*)

DEB

You pooped.

JANET

I pooped? (*she gets hysterical laughing*) I pooped! ...I POOPED!

DEB, TISH, OB, and NURSES

(*everybody starts laughing*)

NURSE ONE

Here comes another one! Ready Janet?

OBSTETRICIAN and TWO NURSE and DEB and TISH

PUSH! ...two, three, four, five, six, seven, eight, nine, ten!
(*overlapping counting*)

DEB and TISH

Come on Janet! Come on! You can do it!

JANET

Grrrrrrrrr...aah! Grrrrrrrrr...aaah!

(*after counting*)
Is the baby okay?

OBSTETRICIAN

Yes!

NURSE TWO

Here comes another contraction, Janet! Ready...

OBSTETRICIAN, TWO NURSE,DEB and TISH

PUSH! …two, three, four, five, six, seven, eight, nine, ten! Come on,

Janet!

(*overlapping counting*)

DEB and TISH

Come on, Janet! You can do it!

(*overlapping counting*)

JANET

Grrrrrrrr...aaah! Is the baby okay? Grrrrrrrr...aaah! Is the baby okay?

OBSTETRICIAN

Yes! Come on, Janet! You can do it!

DEB and TISH

Come on, Janet!!!!!!

OBSTETRICIAN

Here comes another contraction...get ready!

OBSTETRICIAN and TWO NURSES

One, two, three, four, five, six, seven, eight, nine, ten…

OBSTETRICIAN, TWO NURSES and DEB and TISH

PUSH!!!

JANET

Aaaaaaaaaaahh! Is the baby okay?

NURSE ONE

The baby's out!

NURSE TWO

He's out!

DEB

Janet, he's beautiful!

JANET

(*to audience*) A baby came out of me! I couldn't believe it...I also couldn't believe the whole scene. Everyone cheering for me... telling me when to push. It was really fun.

AN ACTOR

Fun?

JANET

Yes, pushing was such a wonderful moment. Deb and Tish cheering me on, my obstetrician screaming like a soccer mom, and two groovy labor and delivery nurses hooting and hollering. They were all so into it. And into me. I was the star.

Scene 8

JILLIAN

One month after I went to Abby's home birth I got pregnant. It was like suddenly I got it! Birth IS normal! (laughs) Now I've never seen a sitcom about that! Can you imagine watching a woman give birth on TV NOT hooked up to machines, with NO doctors and nurses checking everything, and NOT screaming like a wild-woman? Every birth scene I've ever seen on TV is an emergency. No, it's more like a disaster story! The woman and her baby are always on the brink of death – or at least we think they are. Oh! That reminds me of the funniest comedy routine I've ever seen on childbirth! Monty Python's "The Meaning of Life." A pregnant woman is about to have a baby and they're rolling her down the hallway, lots of doors banging open.

ALL ACTORS

(*very loud*) Boom - boom – boom!

JILLIAN

When she gets to the operating room the nurse tells the OBs:

NURSE

(*in a British accent*) The patient is ready!

JILLIAN

and one of the doctors says:

OBSTETRICIAN NUMBER ONE

(*in a British accent*) Alright, very good. Bring the patient into the fetal frightening room!

JILLIAN

The OBs show off their new, very expensive machine that goes:

ALL ACTORS

(*loud*) Ping!

JILLIAN

and everybody claps.

ALL ACTORS

(*clap their hands - quick and very formally*)

JILLIAN

And then after they've assembled a room full of machines the two
OBs look at each other
and say:

OBSTETRICIAN NUMBER TWO

I think we're missing something (*long pause*)…

OBSTETRICIAN NUMBER ONE

Ah, the patient! Yes, the patient!

JILLIAN

and off the nurse goes to find the pregnant woman in labor who is
on a table BEHIND one of the machines! It's just too funny! Oh!
And then, when the woman's pushing her baby out the OB tells her
that she has to listen to him because:

OBSTETRICIAN NUMBER TWO

You're not qualified to deliver your baby!

JILLIAN

Oh boy...not *qualified*?

Scene 9

VOICE OF MIDWIVES

(repeated five times from other actors on stage – voices overlapping each other, each actor starting after the other gets to "hospital." Their voices sound panicked.)

Lisa, you've got to go to the hospital immediately and have a c-section. Call me back.

LISA

(to audience) You'd think I'd have panicked right along with my midwives, but I didn't. I knew the baby's position all the time. I kept telling them the baby was breech!

My take is that the midwives wanted to cover their behinds because every one of them had written down and initialed that the baby had turned head down. But it hadn't turn! Of course they didn't also write in my records that I kept saying I think the baby hasn't turned. I know midwives have techniques for turning babies, but now it was too late in my pregnancy.

AN ACTOR

What did you do?

LISA

I begged them to let me wait and go into labor naturally. Then,
if the baby was breech, fine, do the c-section. But right then I
just felt we had to wait. To me, I was just entering my 40th week.
I knew lots of women carry their first babies longer. I'd done
enough reading to understand that. I was within range. Maybe
my baby was having a hard time turning and maybe he would not
have turned, but let's let HIM decide. It all felt unreal. These were
MIDWIVES! Why weren't they on my side?

Finally, the head midwife called my apartment.

MIDWIFE

Hello. Is this Lisa?

LISA

Yes.

MIDWIFE

Lisa, is somebody with you? Are you alone?

LISA

(*pissed-off tone of voice*) My mother is here.

MIDWIFE

Can you put her on the phone?

LISA

Put her on the phone?

MIDWIFE

Yes, Lisa. I'd like to speak to your mother.

LISA

(to audience) Can you believe they went to my mother? Who did
they think I was – a twelve year old girl?! Justin was out of town
for the day, up in Boston. I wanted him to be with me. I know if
I'd handed the phone to him he'd be on my side. I just needed
someone on my side. But instead I handed the phone to my mother
who later got off the phone with the midwife and grabbed my
hand.

LISA'S MOTHER

Come on, we're going to the hospital.

LISA

When we got to the hospital two midwives met us at the front door.

MIDWIFE ONE

Lisa, we know you're disappointed. We know you wanted a vaginal
delivery.

MIDWIFE TWO

Lisa, you're still a good mother if you don't deliver vaginally.

LISA

(very angry) Good mother? Who said I wasn't a good mother?!
It was the most bizarre experience, people telling me how I was
feeling. I didn't feel disappointed. I just didn't feel a c-section was
called for. My instincts told me to wait, that the baby wasn't fully
cooked – that I should let labor unfold. Maybe a week later I would

have felt panicky and gone for a c-section. But my decision would have been based on whatever communication I was having with the baby. *I* was the mother.

When I got to a room they put an IV in me and shaved me. The midwives were in the room, but really they were useless at this point. I did manage to postpone the c-section as long as I was attached to the fetal heart monitor. The baby's heartbeat was fine. At this point I went through my options. I knew my mother was no help – she was totally stressed out – and Justin was still in Boston unable to get a flight back to me that day. My mother-in-law, who lived in New York and had both her children naturally in the sixties, seemed like the best person to talk to. I knew Paula was on my side. If anyone had any bright ideas it would be her. I opened my cell phone and called Paula.

PAULA

Those midwives aren't worth a damn! Midwives should have known the baby was breech. Good midwives can always tell by looking and touching the stomach.

LISA

I know...I know. But what do I do now? They have me strapped to all these machines.

PAULA

I'll come down there. I will take you out of that hospital...(*pauses*). We can go to Ina May.

LISA

Ina who?

PAULA

The mother of midwifery! Ina May Gaskin at The Farm.

LISA

The Farm?

PAULA

Ina May's birthing center in Tennessee.

LISA

Tennessee? I'M IN WASHINGTON, DC!

PAULA

Really, it's your only option.

LISA

(to audience) Paula was probably right, we should have gone to Tennessee. I should have walked out of there and never walked back. But after I spoke with Paula the nurse came in.

NURSE

We are going to get this baby out. This baby is too big for you to deliver vaginally. It could be nine pounds. You can't birth a nine pound baby.

LISA

I didn't think the baby was that big. Look, I've held a ten pound bag of sugar. I knew I wasn't carrying that kind of weight. I felt like I was in the twilight zone. No one was listening to me. Finally, the nurses and doctors came in and stood against the wall under the clock with their hands crossed.

NURSES AND DOCTORS (*all actors*)
Lisa, we don't know what you're waiting for, but you're going to have a c-section.

LISA
(*very serious tone*) I felt trapped. Of course I wondered why was I being treated like this. Because I'm a woman who's always direct with people? Was I being too bossy? Was it because I was a Black woman and they think I will accept sub-standard care? Maybe when I walked in they thought I didn't have insurance? My mind was going in a thousand directions. But I knew if I was going to get through this I couldn't focus on any of that. They had been mentally working on me for 6 hours. Tennessee was a long ways away. The hospital was making me feel like a negligent mom. Everyone looked at me as if I was crazy for even questioning the c-section. Like, who was *I* to question how much I needed this? They were losing their patience with me.

NURSE
(*annoyed*) It's midnight.

LISA
I decided I could probably only hold them off another hour or two. There was a doctor who could do the c-section right then. In the end, I decided why wait until he was sleep deprived at two in the morning? Do the section.
I was too angry to cry when they wheeled me into the delivery room. I was furious. Pissed off. A nurse was in the room with me.

NURSE

What took you so long? Believe me, it's better to have it come out this way than the other!

LISA

While she was talking all I could think was how cold the room was and how my baby was going to be born into this cold environment.

I held my mother's hand when the section began. When they started I heard the whirr of the instrument cutting me and I could feel tugging. I had to be careful not to look in the glass because then I could see the reflection. Then I could see everything. They had a green partition up so I could disassociate myself from the other half of my body. I felt pulling and tugging and I felt like throwing up. I almost did. The whole lower part of my body was moving back and forth. I heard the "zzz" of the knife and could smell it too. It smelt like lots of blood and burning hair. I kept talking throughout the section because I was so repulsed by the whole thing. I knew if I stopped talking I would be paying attention to the pulling and tugging. As soon as the umbilical cord was cut I heard my baby scream. This is when I began to cry. Ashton was healthy and strong and I was happy in that way that all mothers are happy to know their baby is okay. The nurse made a point of saying –

NURSE

He's certainly breech! Yes, that's a breech baby!

LISA

I wasn't surprised that he was breech. That was never my point.

They gave Ashton to my mother and he stared at me with his big dark eyes. It was a sweet moment. But I couldn't hold him. My guts were totally open. I could still feel the pulling and tugging while they were closing me up. I don't remember a lot more right after that...the recovery room...a puffy pillow with hot air on top of me...I was totally drugged up.

The next morning Justin got a flight back to me and I remember us both crying from the joy of seeing our son together...and the sadness of what I had been through.

You know, after the birth it was hard for me to separate my anger and sadness. I was still furious, but yes, now I was also sad. There was something missing. I felt like my body physically understood that it never went into labor. Like a congested feeling. I had a very strong sense after I had Ashton that my baby had died. Not that I really thought he was dead at any point. I wasn't delusional. I just felt that my body had experienced his birth as a death. My cells, my stomach and my uterus didn't know – aside from my brain – what had happened to the baby. One minute my body was pregnant and the next a knife was put to my stomach and the baby was taken out. As far as my body was concerned there was a big sadness. My body had experienced the birth of my baby as a death.

I never had a labor. I should have been allowed to have at least one labor pain. That's all I wanted.

NURSE
But at least you had a healthy baby!

LISA

Yes, the BABY was healthy. But what about me? What about ME?

Scene 10

JILLIAN

Okay, Okay!...my third birth! Now of course I wanted a homebirth. I tried to do this with a group of fabulous midwives who practiced out of a birth center in south Texas, but their supervising OB would not approve my case for a homebirth or a birth center birth. He said I was this HIGH risk because my birth history wasn't perfect. Basically, I'd never pushed a baby out without drugs. That was enough evidence to declare me unfit for a home birth.

Was I mad? Sure! My only option was the hospital! But this time I wasn't taking any crap.

I did my homework and then I found an OB in town who would help me deliver my baby the way I wanted. But first I made an appointment to interview him.
(*to the doctor*)
What's your episiotomy rate? And your c-section rate? Oh...and just one last question. Do you like women?

OBSTETRICIAN

(*friendly voice with a Southern accent*) In my 30 years practicing medicine I've learned more about birth from laboring women than from medical school.

90

JILLIAN

(*Gets down on her knees like she's thanking God.*) Yes! I'd found an obstetrician in South Texas who believes in birthing women!

On the actual day I gave birth the nurses were baffled! They hadn't seen anything like my birth! A woman giving birth naturally in south Texas? (*bursts out laughing*) Nobody knew what to do!

JILLIAN

(*chanting with midwife by her side*) OOOO...OOOOOO... OOOO...

THREE NURSES

(*mouths all open wide in disbelief*)

JILLIAN

(*louder*) OOOOOOOOO...OOOOOOOOO...OOOOOOOO...

OB

The baby is coming out Jillian!

TWO NURSES

(*Southern accent*) Oh my God! (*one nurse starts to cry*)

JILLIAN

(*to audience*) You know, ALL the hospital staff wanted to hook me up to something. But after a few hours they realized *I* was doing it. Jillian DeMoya was birthing her baby. Me!

I just LOVED everything about going natural...pushing my baby out of my womb...doing it myself...and FEELING my baby pass through me. It was all so exciting, and deeply fulfilling. But what really made the birth extra-special was when my midwife friend took me into the hospital shower *after* the birth and bathed me. In the warm water I felt her hands move gently over my body – like a loving caress. I had never been a part of women caring for each other. It was like all of a sudden my heart was weeping...weeping for joy. I needed this...I needed this experience.

After my third birth I finally got Ina May's words: my body is NOT a lemon.

Scene 11

SANDY

Hi mom, it's Sandy.

SANDY'S MOTHER

Yes, dear. How are you feeling?

SANDY

Not great. That doctor...

SANDY'S MOTHER

(*angry*) ...is good for nothing! If I ever see him again I might hurt him!

SANDY

Me too.

Mom...

SANDY'S MOTHER

Yes?

SANDY

(*hesitant voice*) Tina just had her baby last night... at a birth center...in water.

SANDY'S MOTHER

(*horrified*) In water?! You mean in a bath tub?

SANDY

A birthing pool. I was there...she had her baby under candlelight... with midwives.

SANDY'S MOTHER

(*even more horrified reaction*) Midwives!

SANDY

It's not crazy to give birth with midwives, mom. It's not, like, midwives are some hippies who deliver babies in cornfields in Iowa.

SANDY'S MOTHER

I didn't say that, Sandra.

SANDY

Then why do you sound so alarmed? At Tina's birth her midwife was there for her every step of the labor, telling her she was going to be alright.

MIDWIFE

(*intense, passionate*) You can do it, Tina. You ARE doing it!

TINA

Aaaaaaah! That hurt like hell!

MIDWIFE

(*happy, passionate, encouraging*) Great! That's EXACTLY how it's supposed to feel!

SANDY

Wow. I mean, *that's exactly how it's supposed to feel?*! It hurt like hell and that's OKAY? When I yelled out during MY labor all I remember is a nurse asking me -

NURSE

(*friendly*) Ready for your epidural?

SANDY

I had no idea a woman didn't have to be rescued from pain. You know, mom, I used to hear the word "midwife" and think, like, the baby's going to be born out on the bedroom floor. Now I think... what's so weird about that?

SANDY'S MOTHER

What about the safety of the baby, Sandra?

SANDY

Of the BABY! What about the mother?

SANDY'S MOTHER

Of course the mother's safety is important. But…having a baby in
water! Sandra, be serious about your birth. Stop fooling around.

SANDY

Fooling around? Is wanting something different next time fooling
around? I don't know…I just don't know…I mean…all I do know
is that if I have another baby I really want to push my baby out
vaginally with only close friends and candlelight and maybe even in
water. It's not, like, THAT stupid.

SANDY'S MOTHER

You had so much trouble the first time, Sandra. Do you really want
to risk it?

SANDY

(*to the audience. Sandy starts getting emotional*) Okay.. if my
mother really didn't want me to do it... I mean…if she's really
not comfortable with it then... maybe .. no midwives…no
candlelight…no water... for my mother…for her.. maybe I'd do it in
a hospital again. It's... just one day.

Scene 12

JILLIAN

Okay!...birth number four! So fun...so communal...so NOT Desi

Arnez and Lucy running around frantic shouting:

DESI and LUCY

It's time!

JILLIAN

That was my first birth. "Birth As Entertainment." I was SO over that. This birth was about showing up.

After giving birth naturally in the hospital with my third child all of a sudden I was now no longer this HIGH risk. I was practically peeing in my pants! I could have a homebirth! Home...midwives... doulas... girlfriends. Oh, yes, and Ramone, my husband! I wanted him there too! But it was great to see him finally understand that what I needed to give birth was a solid team of women. Okay! Here was my team! Carla, my midwife, Diana, my doula, Patty, my friend who is a nurse, and Nancy, a girlfriend who loves me the most in life. I wanted everyone at my birth to be significant.

And the birth itself? Labor started at around 3am – just a "funny," uncomfortable feeling I took a bath while everyone was sleeping. In the morning, the contractions were really much the same – just this "funny" feeling. I made banana bread while the kids ate breakfast. I loved that my kids could be at my birth! To prepare them we watched a lot of birth videos and did some role playing. I'd say, "You know, it's going to sound like this –

(*very* loud, but not panicked, scream) "AAAAAAA-HA!" And then they'd copy that noise back to me:

JILLIAN'S THREE BOYS

(*loud, deep sound, but not panicked scream*) Aaaaaaah...ha!

JILLIAN

Now, you do it! Ready? (*she gets the audience to repeat the sound back*)

AUDIENCE

Aaaaaaaaaaaaaa...ha!

JILLIAN

We had a great laugh!

Okay! This is just so much fun to talk about! My contractions really got going around 7pm. Whew! Were they painful...the pain went from my uterus down the tops of my thighs. Diana suggested I get into our tub filled with warm water.

(*Jillian stands up and walks to the chair next to her – she's walking into her birth story. Seven actors have gotten up from their chairs and surround Jillian - Diana is the closest to her.*)

I stepped into the tub...and then sat in the water.

(*she slouches down like she's lying in a tub. Diana sits down next to her. You can see the relief on Jillian's face. Then she bursts out laughing*).

(*very loud and enthusiastic*) Oh, Diana! We have got to spread the word about water!

97

(her sounds are low and slow) Ooooooo…Oooooooo…Oooooooo…

(The actors gather around Jillian. Her contractions are intense. She's loud, but not hysterical.)

Here comes another one…Aaaaaaaaaaaaah…Aaaaaaaaaaaah Aaaaaaaaaaaah…

ALL ACTORS
(softly) You can do it, Jillian! You can do it! You CAN do it!

JILLIAN
(softly) Here's another…Aaaaaaaaaaaaah…

ALL ACTORS
(softly) You're doing everything right…you're doing everything right…

JILLIAN
(breathing softly, but with intensity) I'm hungry…

DIANA
What do you want?

JILLIAN
Scrambled eggs…I need scrambled eggs!

(to audience) I just love that I ate scrambled eggs at 8 centimeters! Why not?! I was hungry. Simple. Not complicated. Home was SO not complicated. Ten minutes after I ate the eggs my body was

ready to push.

(birthing)

MIDWIFE

Go ahead and push, Jillian.

JILLIAN

I can push? Where?

MIDWIFE

Where ever YOU want.

JILLIAN

(to audience) I could push ANYWHERE I wanted to! Isn't that great?!! I definitely wanted to stay IN the birthing pool.

(Back to Jillian's birth. Her birth sounds are powerful, deep. The birth scene is not chaotic, but instead warm, quiet, loving)

JILLIAN

Aaaaaaaaaaaaaah…Aaaaaaaaaaaaah....Aaaaaaaaaaaaah…

MIDWIFE

You're doing great, Jillian!

JILLIAN'S CHILD

(high-pitched child's voice) Good job, mommy!

JILLIAN

(louder sounds...keeps making sounds while others talk)

Aaaaaaaaaaaaah….Aaaaaaaaaaaah…Aaaaaaaaaaaaaaaaaaaaah…

DIANA

Jillian, you're almost there!

NANCY

You can do it, Jillian!

JILLIAN'S HUSBAND

I love you, Honey! You're beautiful!

PATTY

You *are* doing it!

JILLIAN

Aaaaaaaaaaaaah…Aaaaaaaaaaaah….Aaaaaaaaaaaah…

MIDWIFE

Good job, Jillian!

PATTY

This is SO great –

JILLIAN'S HUSBAND

You can do it, Honey!

JILLIAN'S CHILD

Mommy, I can see the head!

MIDWIFE

Do you want to feel her head, Jillian?

JILLIAN

Yes! YES! *(she puts her hand at the open)*...Ooooooo…it hurts! It hurts so much!

MIDWIFE

Good!

JILLIAN

(Jillian's hands are still down. She looks orgasmic, a big grin on her face, then she copies Abby's birth sound)

WAAAA-HOO!....Waaaa-hooo!...Waaaaa-hooo!

MIDWIFE

Here she comes!

JILLIAN'S CHILD

Her head has lots of hair!

JILLIAN

I want to catch her! *(feels baby's head with her hand)* Is that her?

MIDWIFE

Yes! Now, push slowly, Jillian... Push as slow as possible.

JILLIAN

(slow, steady pushing)

Aaaaaaaaaaaaah…Aaaaaaaaaaaah....Aaaaaaaaaaaaaaaaaaaaaaaaaaaa aaaaaaaaaaaaaaaaaaaaaaah! Ooooooooooooh! It BURNS! It BURNS!

MIDWIFE

Great! Here she comes!

JILLIAN

(starts to cry)

DIANA

She's out! She's out!

JILLIAN'S CHILD

(kneels down at the opening to Jillian's vulva) She's beautiful, mommy! She's an angel!

JILLIAN HUSBAND

(crying) You did it, Honey...YOU did it!

JILLIAN

I DID IT! *I did it… (a tender moment of hugging and crying. Birth team surrounds Jillian, hugging her, looking proud of her)*

(after Jillian takes her moment…actors say slowly)

AMANDA

I did it!

JANET

I did it.

VANESSA

I did it.

SANDY

I did it.

BETH

I did it.

LISA

I did it.

NATALIE

I did it.

End of Act 2

Postscript

Sandy decided for her second birth she wanted to delivery vaginally. At her 36 week check-up her obstetrician said to her, "This is going to be a big baby." After hearing that she walked out, switched to hospital-based midwives and had a drug-free vaginal birth with a midwife and doula by her side.

Natalie had her second baby at home in water unassisted with only her husband, girlfriend and daughter present. She went for no prenatal care.

Beth had her second baby by planned c-section. She has no regrets.

Vanessa had her second baby in the hospital with an epidural. She tore again.

Janet had no more children.

With the threat of being induced with drugs at 36 weeks pregnant because she may be developing pre-eclampsia **Lisa** decided to naturally induce herself at home. Several days later she went into labor and gave birth in a hospital naturally to her son, Casper, with her partner and a midwife by her side.

Jillian moved with her husband and 4 children back to the Midwest to be closer to family. She went on to become a doula and hopes to be a midwife one day.

Amanda had her second baby naturally at a birth center with midwives. She chanted "My body rocks!" throughout her labor.

PHOTOS

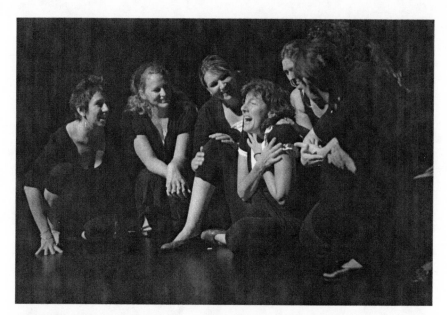

Chicago, Illinois performance, BOLD 2007 / photo credit: Anita Evans

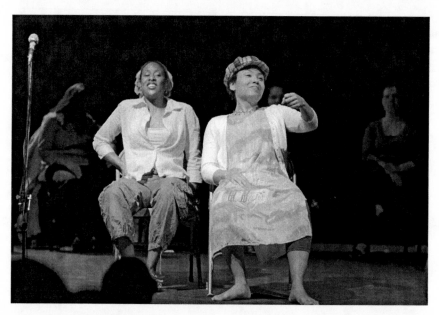

Boston, Massachusetts performance, 2007 / photo credit: Kim Indresano

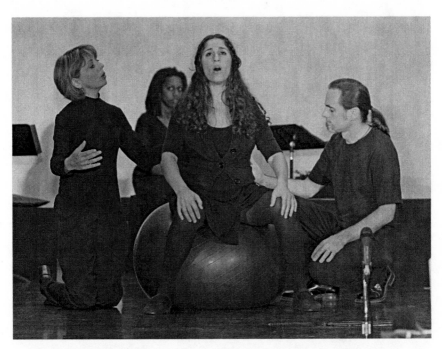

Santa Rosa, California, BOLD 2007 / photo credit: Ananda Fierro

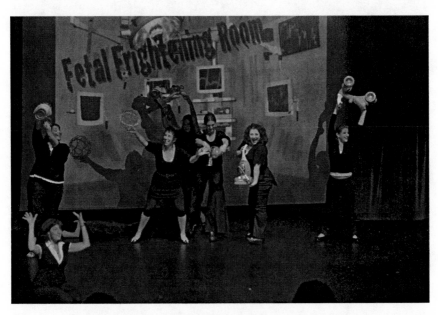

Chicago, Illinois, BOLD 2007 / photo credit: Anita Evans

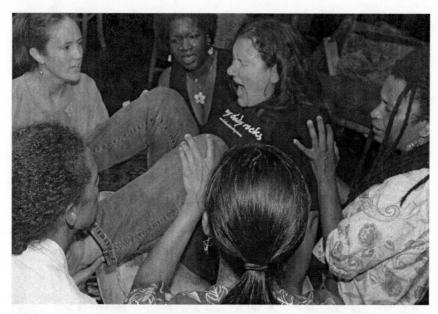

Maui, Hawaii, BOLD 2007 / photo credit: www.tommckinlayphotography.com

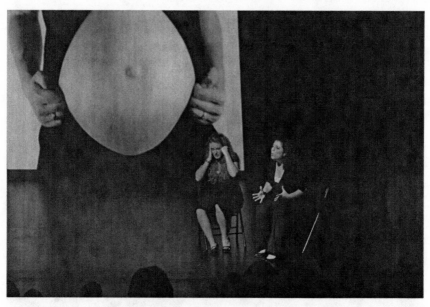

Chicago, Illinois, BOLD 2007 / photo credit: Anita Evans

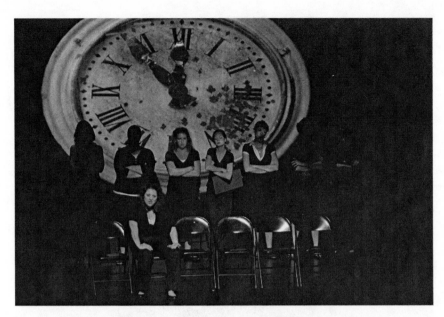

Chicago, Illinois, BOLD 2007 / photo credit: Anita Evans

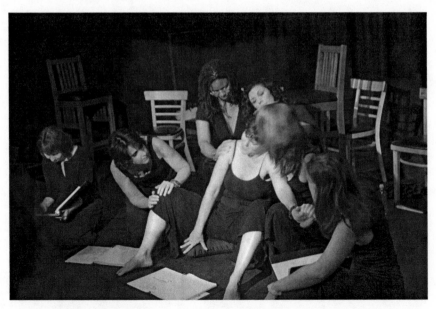

11.BOLD Austin, Texas, BOLD 2007 / photo credit: Nancy Joe

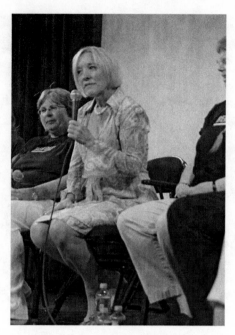

Dr. Christiane Northrup, BOLD 2006 Talkback, New York City / photo credit: www.jfwphotography.com

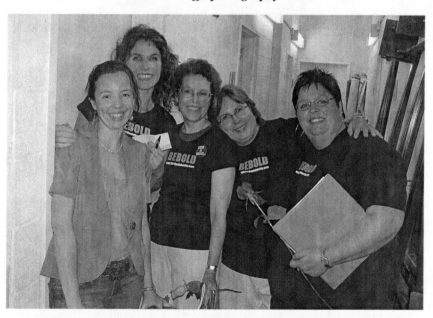

Backstage, BOLD 2006, New York City.
(from left to right) Heidi Miami-Marshall, Karen Brody, Henci Goer,
Barbara Harper, Jillian DeMoya (yes, the real Jillian!)

*After*BIRTH: Playwright's Notes

After people see the play I get asked all the time two things: why is the play so against the medical community and why is the play so anti-midwife? It's amusing to me to see how a play can be perceived in two polar opposite ways.

I can understand feeling that this play is anti-medical. While I never set out to write a play that was against the medical community my one commitment when I wrote the play was to tell the truth. It became difficult to tell the truth about how low-risk women are giving birth in America and not find at the end a negative picture was being painted of the medical establishment. The truth is that over one-third of women are getting cesareans in America, nearly all women are requesting epidurals and few are giving birth without drugs. Anyone who has studied the effects of drug intervention on mothers giving birth will know that it is common for one intervention to lead to another. In real life when I listened to women tell me their birth stories this is the story I heard over and over again. Many women who wanted epidurals, like the character Sandy, had no idea that an epidural could cause a fever in her and the baby and that it would often require another drug to move the labor along. This is the reality of childbirth inside most hospitals today.

I do find it interesting right after the play when audience members tell me there was no woman who had a positive experience with her obstetrician. This is not true. Janet's story is actually one of a woman who found herself a great support team and her doctor was "screaming like a soccer mom" right by her side. She loved her obstetrician – which is what some women I interviewed told me. What I want people to get in a story like Janet's is that she chose to have an epidural and it went well, but the fact that it went well (despite a brief medical scare) had very much to do with the support she had.

Am I promoting epidurals in this play? This is what one childbirth professional expressed to me when she read the play and counted the word epidural eighty-seven times (I haven't counted!). Again, my answer goes back to telling the truth. Most women are having epidurals – that's the truth - so it wasn't surprising to me to know that epidural was mentioned so much in the play. I'm at peace with it.

What I am less happy about is that some midwives do not like the play. I am a strong supporter of the midwifery model of care and while I know many midwives work hard to bring this kind of care into the hospital setting another part of me – the playwright seeking truth – heard from a significant number of women who did not have positive experiences with midwives in hospitals. What always gets to me when I hear negative birth stories with hospital-based midwives is that many of these mothers, and especially their friends and families, think midwifery care failed them. What I want women to know is that seeing a midwife in a hospital does not guarantee you midwifery care. While there are midwives practicing midwifery care in hospitals today it often takes great communication between the midwife and the hospital to dance around the delicate balance of offering a style of care in an institution that is not set up to support that type of care.

I am saddened every time I hear a birth story of a woman seeing a hospital-based midwife who goes into labor, develops a minor complication and due to hospital protocols she no longer qualifies (in the medical model's eyes) for midwifery care. This is a highly-charged issue in midwifery, one that doesn't have an easy solution because the reality is that most women give birth in hospitals so midwives are desperately needed there.

The question for women who want a gentle drug-free birth with a hospital-based midwife to think about is: are most of the women using this midwife having low/no intervention births? In some communities the answer is yes, in others it is not. This is where connecting to the existing birth community is crucial to learn what options exists in your area.

I have also heard whisperings that a play about childbirth should only include positive birth stories. To this I again come back to the truth. That is not the truth about childbirth today. The play I wanted to write was about the truth. I do think it's important to tell positive birth stories, but when I wrote *Birth* I decided this play was about telling the truth about childbirth so that a collective healing and sisterhood could take place among women who have given birth. To me healing and sisterhood are two crucial ingredients to improving childbirth today. These two powerful forces allow us to move towards a childbirth solution that is women-centered. We can't just go from crisis to solution. There are too many of these mothers who are injured from their birth experiences. They must be heard – and healed. And alongside them, like in the play with Jillian and Amanda's births, we must also hear from our sisters who are having powerful birth experiences so that they can teach us how they got there; show us the way.

Did you notice that the character Jillian is really the spine of the play? I hope so! When I called Jillian to interview her about her birth experiences she had such a magnetic personality. I've never heard a funnier laugh. She has one of those laughs that gets the whole room laughing. I think we spoke for four hours! I knew I wanted to use her story in the play, but I never thought she'd be so central to what the play is all about. Jillian's story is about hope. Her character is about making right what was wrong. And she's about a woman who works hard to release her "birth baggage" and become more connected to herself. Once this is in place, not too surprisingly, her powerful birth is possible at the end of the play.

If there is anywhere in the play where I'm preaching I feel Jillian's final birth is it. To end the play with such a powerful birth was my way of putting out there that having a pleasurable birth is not only possible, but necessary for women. Accessing pleasure always takes you to a better place. Amanda knew this in her birth when she shouted "My Body Rocks!" and Jillian showed this in her final birth - that after two disappointing births she too could have a "My Body Rocks" birth experience.

I love Amanda in the play. Her "My Body Rocks!" mantra conveys the power of the mind when you're giving birth. She had a hospital birth, but knew that the best thing she could do was to stay home until late in her labor with a doula and keep her mind positive. It's the law of attraction. A positive mind towards childbirth attracts a positive birth experience. Amanda didn't just repeat "My Body Rocks!" she believed it in her gut.

Beth, the planned c-section story, was by far the most passionate c-section story I'd heard. I included her not just because she planned her c-section, but I thought her reasons were fascinating. Even though a planned c-section would not be my choice for giving birth I understood Beth's reasoning. She didn't want to be induced and she knew most women were. She didn't want an episiotomy and she noticed many women got it. The one part that was hard for me to include was her mis-information, specifically her fear of incontinence. Studies don't support that women who give birth vaginally have a greater risk of incontinence. But I kept it in there because this is exactly what I found many women who are fearful of childbirth do. They find anything to support their point regardless of the validity. Beth was certainly that character although I must say I so enjoyed speaking with her. It was often hard to get women to be honest with me about their birth experiences, but not Beth!

Vanessa and Sandy were perhaps the most typical birth stories I heard. Vanessa, who felt her birth experience was good, spent the day hooked up to machines with her family watching television. When she told me her story I remembered the first birth I ever saw on TLC's *A Baby's Story* and how floored I was that the woman had been given an epidural and everyone was watching television as she labored. I wanted to show through Vanessa's story this culture of disconnection that I feel is so prevalent in childbirth, and our society, today.

In both Vanessa and Sandy's births they were most definitely not the center of their birth experiences. Sandy's was a tragic story of an educated woman who walked into the hospital and felt like she had stepped onto an out-of-control freight train. Oh, how often I heard this story. While I was moved by so many stories there were a few – like Sandy's – that after I hung up the phone I wept. When she told me how she hugged her mother after the birth and cried it brought to life for me the tragic scene of a grown woman giving birth unsupported and then regressing to a child who desperately needed her mother.

Sandy was a clear example of how one intervention can lead to another. She represented the woman who lost her connection to her intuitive self almost from the time she got pregnant. Her postpartum experience was not included in the original version of the play, but I added it because when I spoke with Sandy after she read the play she reminded me how much her postpartum was a part of her birth experience. I thought adding her postpartum period really made it clear to women that birth is NOT "just one day." I also wanted to highlight the complications that can arise from a cesarean, another story I heard from alot mothers.

Lisa's story was also heartbreaking and yet I felt it was necessary. In Lisa's story I wanted to show that even a strong woman has a hard time challenging the medical system. I also wanted to show the profound affect a cesarean can have on a woman. It was a hard choice to let Lisa tell very graphic details of her cesarean, but I felt her words were so precise and charged with emotion. Lisa really takes us into the operating room by describing her sensations. And then to hear a mother say the birth of her baby felt like a death….well, it really drives home just how traumatic a cesarean can be for a woman.

The play was originally seven stories when it premiered in 2005. The eighth story – Natalie – was written in 2007. I had wanted to write a story about a woman who had a forced episiotomy. I had heard this story too many times yet I didn't interview a woman whose story seemed right for the play. When I met Natalie at a BOLD Red Tent in New York City in September 2006 I knew I had my story. She was so beautiful, inside and out, and so full of trust in her body and the birth process. To end up with a forced episiotomy showed just how much any woman can be violated when she is giving birth. She said no and was still cut. That's sexual violation. To me Natalie's story and her decision to birth her second baby at home unassisted without any prenatal care positions childbirth today firmly on the women's rights agenda. Is this what women today have to do to get a powerful, respected birth?

On a lighter note, cast members from past productions have often asked me what lines in the play stand out to me. Here are a few:

"I finally began to walk through all my birth baggage."

Jillian, Act 2, scene 5

"Waa-hoo!"

Abby, the woman Jillian watches giving birth at home, Act 2, scene 5

"Waa-hoo!"

Jillian copying Abby's ecstatic birth sound during her 4th birth, Act 2, scene 12

"I thought the birth was just one day. How bad can it be to be around someone you don't like for one day?"

Sandy, Act 1, scene 3

"How's a baby going to get out of such a narrow space?"

Janet, Act 1, scene 3

"I'll come down there. I will take you out of that hospital. We can go to Ina May. We can go to The Farm."

Paula, Act 2, scene 9

"My body had experienced the birth of my baby as a death."

Lisa, Act 2, scene 9

"YOU'RE IN THE HAPPIEST PLACE IN THE HOSPITAL. THE MATERNITY WARD! WHY ARE YOU NOT HAPPY?!!!"

Sandy, Act 1, scene 7

"My vagina will NEVER be the same."

Natalie, Act 2, scene 6

"I didn't want a midwife. I wasn't going to deliver in the bath water!"

Beth, Act 1, scene 3

"How could I forget a sensation that felt like the baby was coming out of my butt?"

Vanessa, Act 1, scene 3

"WOW, I mean, that's exactly how it's supposed to feel? It hurt like hell and that's okay?"

Sandy, Act 2, scene 11

"Oh, Diana! We have got to spread the word about water!"

Jillian, Act 2, scene 12

"I just love that I ate scrambled eggs at 8 centimeters!"

Jillian, Act 2, scene 12

And of course:

"My Body Rocks!"

Amanda, Act 1, scene 10

Truth was my guide as I wrote this play. My hope is that in the years to come a new truth about childbirth emerges, one with every mother at the center of her birth experience, getting her needs met, knowing her body rocks. In short: pleasurable births for all women!

I believe the pendulum is swinging and this vision – of childbirth and pleasure - will emerge in the years to come.

Rock on, BOLD warriors.

BOLD

Emails and Stories

BOLD feedback from audience

Dear Janet, Divya, Nidhi, Vasanti, Estelle, Elisha, Amy, Lola, Anju, Melissa,

BRAVO! BRAVA! You did it! A staging of *Birth* over the Labour Day weekend in consonance with performances worldwide.

I found the writing really riveting. Far from being scary or gory or a turnoff in any way, it was great to hear about the diversity of experiences. The intimate setting worked really well and all the performers seemed to be really into their roles.

At the end of the evening, my mind was echoing with the chorus "MY BODY ROCKS" and I left feeling quite envious of my dog Madonna and every other mama who's been through the bold birth experience.

Three cheers for you all. Well done!

- Punita, New Delhi, India, BOLD 2006

Thank you so much for a very thought-provoking, informative, AND entertaining evening last night! There were some fine actors on that stage..as well as heart-felt. And the thoughtful questions and discussion that followed was also outstanding. You know, pioneers in beginning new things do tend to be women who recognize their "bodies rock" and are not afraid to misbehave just slightly. Kudos to you!

- Audience member, former obstetric nursing professor, Lynchburg, Virginia, BOLD 2006

I had to email when I got home to thank you. The reason I wanted to thank you is because I appreciated the play but most importantly the experience. Each story was well done but the stories I related to about natural childbirth brought me back to a time of strength and empowerment. I especially realized its importance during the discussion time. During the play there were times that I couldn't stop crying. I was crying because I am not so sure I realized what I did as a woman. Thank you for letting me be in that space again. I don't know if this is corny - or even makes sense for that matter - but I really connected to the strength that's inside me and that the people surrounding me support that strength. Amanda's "My Body Rocks" story was particularly familiar. I also remembered what a great time I had giving birth to both of my children. I think I am going to sit them down and tell them their birth stories and tell them over and over again.

- Audience member, New York City, BOLD 2006

This is my forth time I've seen "Birth." I like to keep coming to see what I learn and honestly to reconnect with other people that come to the performances.

I am again reminded of the dismissal disempowering state of the majority of maternity care in the United States. Of instincts being shut down, of mothers not being supported. I hope this play can help women stand up.

- Amy, certified nurse midwife, Chicago, BOLD 2007

I very much enjoyed the performance Saturday night, and I also appreciate all the effort gone to produce 'Birth.' The performance seemed to be very successful and well-received, and the collective enthusiasm of audience, actors and panel participants was encouraging and very powerful.

I opened a solo OB-Gyn office after realizing there was a real niche for a small practice that could provide more personalized care for women. I also realized that I wouldn't want to go to an OB office that had five or six delivery doctors, so why not practice the way I would want if I were a patient?

- OB-GYN, Asheville, North Carolina BOLD 2006

Best 20 bucks I've spent in awhile ... it was super to be watching the spirits of these actresses share the greater birth story. I was moved over and over again. Recalling my own 3 birth experiences and feeling deeply blessed for my stories of each birth. My heart goes out to women worldwide who don't have this experience of a blissful easy birth. I now have a deeper empathy. Thanks for bringing it home.

- Audience member, Maui BOLD 2007

Loved Vagina Monologues, wanted to experience this. I came away thinking that I was not alone in the losing control of my birthing. I thought the MD's were GODS. Thank you for pointing us towards our birth sovereignty. Thank you women who showed us to take back our natural rights.

- Audience member, Maui, BOLD 2007

BOLD organizers speak

From BOLD Maui, Hawaii...

Well ladies and gentlemen ... we did it. We rocked Maui. Our three performances were phenomenal, if I have to say so myself. At the first performance there were over 200 people in attendance. The audience, laughed, cried and were with us in every moment. We got a standing ovation at the end. Midwives came from the outer islands. Tears of joy streamed down my face as we went off the stage for the last time ...we did it, we did it, we DID it! The Maui News (our biggest newspaper) has made us the Feature of the Week for our September 15th show. Another newspaper did an Arts and Entertainment feature on us.

You would think I would be exhausted after our second performance ... especially since there was a talkback after the show and we had to move all of the furniture out of the theatre when we were done but .... there I was, up at 1:49am, typing the Maui report to other BOLD Organizers. At this show there were 166 tickets sold ... for Maui on a Saturday night for BIRTH, these are fabulous numbers. The show tonight had a different crowd. Last week, the midwives from all of the island came. This time, the crowd was a diverse group of teenagers, pregnant moms, infants, older people ...

people of all ages and stages ... they totally rode the waves with us and it was spectacular.

One of our actresses presented us with gifts during intermission ... a scrapbook ... one page for each of us with pictures she has taken along the way. We each signed each other's books like a yearbook. What a fabulous idea.

And one of my best moments? When my 13 year old son said "mom ... I really didn't want to go see it but ... it was awesome!!!! I want to come see it again."

After the final show we had an "after-BIRTH" party that was outrageous ... Indian, Ethiopian and Jamaican food (which totally sold out) and music from our local Marimba ensemble ... out of this world. The after-Birth was located in a Market less than 2 minutes away from the theatre, as soon as we were exiting the theatre the music drew us there. The proprietor of the marketplace said he had never seen anything like it.

Thanks to all for the journey ... and thank you Karen Brody for helping bring the consciousness of all beings to a higher level. You are da bomb!!!!! This is an unbelievable project and I feel so very blessed to be a part of it. Thank you, thank you, thank you!

With lots of love from paradise!

-      Robin Garrison BOLD 2007 Organizer in Maui, Hawaii

From BOLD Flagstaff, Arizona

We had a beautiful two day blessing way! The night before the show after rehearsal we had one of the moms share her birth story and then everybody stayed for another hour and a half having our own little talkback and discussion. Earlier that night I also had everybody choose 10 beautiful glass beads - one for themselves, one for their children, their beloved, for sadness they felt, for forgiveness, for their body, for their own mother, their grandchildren to be, for the way they make a difference in the world and one for The Great Mother. (Not necessarily in that order). I collected each person's beads and on Saturday strung them together on a wire that they could "use" for meditation, while nursing, etc. Each individual string of beads contained a large red glass heart at one end - showing that although we each are so unique we all share a spark of the Great Heart. After a silly and fun warm-up, we had a beautiful circle before the show on Saturday and I gave each person their string of beads. It was really special to all of us. OH! And on the night before when we were choosing beads the pregnant mommy in the cast ("Sandy") felt her baby move for the first time!! And it wasn't a gas bubble! She burst into tears and so did the rest of us!

And on the performance night:

Oh my…it was an incredible night. The show was received with so much love and support. Not a dry eye in the house throughout - lots of verbal support from the audience. Standing ovation and all. We did a staged reading and the cast consisted of mostly beginning actors - all of them mothers. Every one of these actors were great. I was the proud parent, a giddy girlfriend, and a humbled director the evening of our performance and throughout the rehearsal process.

I was an actress, director, etc, in New York for many years and when I moved to Flagstaff and became a mother, I felt ready to hang up those former hats. I willingly embraced my role as mother and shifted my "career focus" to teaching yoga, doing occasional commercials when they come up, and being the go-to gal in Flagstaff for Bradley families and prenatal yoga. I NEEDED to produce/direct *Birth* because it seemed to be the right thing to do - and I knew how to do it.

When I came upstairs from the theatre basement on our performance evening after leading the warm-up and blessingway for the cast - the sound of a full house of people talking and anticipating the show - stopped me dead in my tracks. I burst into tears. My stage manager was a little worried for a second! But for me, it was a moment of complete confirmation that everything I'm doing right now is exactly what I should be doing. It all felt so easy and so right to be combining my love of mommies, my love of teaching, and my love of theatre into one perfect moment.

Congratulations to everybody!! What an incredible project and circle of women to be a part of. I envisioned with our cast the other night that our little circle of ripples in Flagstaff kept expanding and expanding until it met the ripples of the cast in Seattle and Chicago and Boston etc etc etc. It was so beautiful to think of all of you that night.

- Mary Denmead, BOLD 2007 Organizer, Flagstaff, Arizona

PS - Heard a great birth story from one of my Bradley students today - She was "due" next week - water broke at 39 weeks, she labored beautifully at home the next morning, her and her husband danced and moaned through every contraction, stood forehead to forehead the whole way -she went from 5-10 centimeters in an hour (go momma!) and her husband caught the baby with midwives quietly observing. So beautiful! Let's all have what she got!

Two days before show time for BOLD Pensacola, Florida...

Hi ladies... I'm finally taking a few minutes to BREATHE.

First, let me say – I've never in my life said I wanted a Prozac - and I think I've reached that point! If this is transition - I think I want the epidural!!! But, like birth, when it's this difficult - it means it's almost over.

And on opening night:

TONIGHT IS OPENING NIGHT! The first of 6 shows across the panhandle of Florida. I'm practically peeing in my pants (can you tell I've got the lines of Jillian nearly memorized as well!?).

I keep trying to do deep breaths, my best friend is a chiropractor and has given me some whole food supplements for the adrenal glands to help lol. That was her "gift" to me in preparation for the play a couple days ago.

I'm so thrilled. So far, this has already sparked quite a stir in our community. I think - no I KNOW - that women WILL BE TOUCHED and moved by this. In a positive way. Change WILL happen in our area from this. Perhaps slowly, but surely.

I love the fact that were the talk of the town right now. I have people, including cast, saying that this is the most talked about show that they've ever been involved in or seen! That just BLOWS MY MIND! Now I just hope we get a turnout to reflect that!! With 6 shows, we NEED warm bodies in those seats!!!

And I'm also thrilled that 4 of our shows are on a college campus. Students are finally back in town. We may go do some ticket giveaways on campus depending on the turnout from this weekend. Of course, ticket sales are important, but getting young college women - the women who CAN Make a difference - who still have time to stand up & let their voices be heard and who are still the consumers, it's EXTREMELY important. I think we may give the whole freaking nursing dept free tickets!!!

I also have been very impressed - so far my phone is ringing off the hook, the birthing centers phone is ringing off the hook - people wanting info about the play, how to get there, can tickets be bought at the door. A large number of men, and even older women (we have a large senior citizen community - I mean, we ARE Florida you know!).

I really believe that in addition to being an educational and entertaining show, this can be a healing opportunity. For SO many women.

My brain is obviously going a million miles a minute. I'll calm it down eventually - probably not till tomorrow.
So - I would say wish us luck, but that's bad luck - so wish us to break a leg!

And the second night:

When the second performance began we all reflected on the last 9 weeks back stage. We laughed, we cried, we got our final jitters as we did our usual warm up.

On stage we go...we ROCKED the house. We had 30 labor and delivery nurses attend from the local hospital that had refused to endorse us. (Turns out a lactation consultant snuck a poster into the nurses break room without the nurse manager knowing). How wonderful to see the internal rebellion!!!!!!

- Angela Dowling, BOLD 2007 Organizer, Pensacola, Flordia

From BOLD Boston, Massachusetts...

It's hard to imagine that all those months of planning are over in one fell swoop! Julie in Chicago made the perfect analogy that for us organizers, our BOLD events are just like a wedding reception – so many people to talk to, moments to capture, details to attend to, trying to do it all yet not miss being in the moment...so much planning and preparation, and then when it's finally over you can't believe it all went by so quickly. I keep asking...do I get to take the honeymoon?

Back in January, shortly after I signed on as a BOLD organizer, one of my childhood friends dropped dead from a heart attack. He was 37 years old.

I have a sign on my desk that says *"What would you attempt to do if you knew you could not fail?"* Rob's death made me less fearful of failing in many aspects of my life, and was a huge reminder that we never know what life has in store for us. I decided I was going to be really BOLD and go for it, even if it didn't work out exactly as I planned.

And in some ways, it didn't. I never expected to feel so connected to and inspired by a group of women I had never met before. I never expected to make some wonderful new friends, who began this journey with me as BOLD Boston volunteers, and ended it as friends. And the nicest surprise I never expected – having Karen as the guest of honor for both our BOLD Red Tent event and our Saturday evening performance of *Birth*!

Some other things didn't go as planned, and not in a good way. We lost our first director, and then brought on another director who was truly difficult to work with and in the end did not capture the essence of the play in some ways. We were really surprised by the lack of volunteer support we received from our local doula/CBE/midwifery community (they did support us in other ways, just not in the ways we expected, and really could have used more help in the planning stages). Our matinee performance had low attendance (though those 50-60 people may not have seen the show if it was only 2 evenings). And who knew it was going to be in the 80's and humid on one of the last days of September in Boston, making it very, very hot in our non-air conditioned theatre!

However, overall I'd say our BOLD events were quite a success! It looks like we raised between $12 - $14,000. We comped more seats than expected (though weren't even able to give seats away to OB's – we had 40 set aside for OB's, and not one took us up on free tickets!) and we had really expected sponsorship that just didn't happen, as much as we tried. Still, we reached about 500 people with the BOLD message. We had requests from Simmons College, Boston University and Harvard to bring the play there.

And there were other highlights. It was wonderful to have the "real" Sandy in the audience and on our Talkback panel. She was truly moved by the performance. One of the actresses left me a message that said it was "honestly one of the best times of my life"– this from a spirited Italian woman who clearly loves life – that message alone makes it all worth it! And to top it off, it was incredibly rewarding to exercise my brain in a way it hasn't been in my 4.5 years as a stay at home mother!

Thank you all for walking this journey with me! I loved collaborating with all of you and hearing all of your wonderful ideas and feeling your support from hundreds and thousands of miles away. I loved being part of a tribe of warm, thoughtful, caring, intelligent and hard-working women! I loved being BOLD with all of you!!!

- Cathleen Barstow, Boston, Massachusetts, BOLD 2007

From BOLD Hartford, Connecticut in 2006...

My mother – who directed the play - says she is still "high" from the weekend. And I am at a loss for words to describe the many things I feel about being a part of BOLD in its first year. I am proud, humbled, in awe of the women involved in this project and so much more.

September, 2007:

I feel like, to me, organizing BOLD takes place on two levels - educating the public on a large scale, and having this intimate, bonding, growing experience on a small scale with the actresses. Each part of the process needs to be nurtured in a different way, but both parts are vital to the success of the project

- Michal Klau-Stevens, BOLD Organizer 2006 and 2007, Hartford, Connecticut

From BOLD India...

It was fantastic, amazing, magic! Wonderful really--thanks so much for writing it Karen....words fail me here....truth.

I usually am not at a loss for words, but in the days after our BOLD performance I have been thinking (really feeling) about our intense and joyous times with the play. So many people have expressed appreciation and admiration for the quality of the performance--and it is truly amazing that we were able to do what we did, and bond the way we did. Each and every one stepped into the characters and brought them alive spectacularly. Reminds me of an old bumper sticker--"The goddess is alive and magic is afoot."

And there, in the background, was Divya, midwife-ing it all with her enthusiasm. "You can do it." "We can do it!"

- Janet Chawla, BOLD 2006 Organizer, New Delhi, India

From BOLD Austin, Texas in 2006...

It was such an honor to perform this and bring it to Austin this year. As a co-director I couldn't have asked for a better performance. As an actress I was honored to portray Jillian and be amongst the other women as they brought their characters to life. It was all so moving, and deeply fulfilling to quote Jillian.

Karen, this play and this BOLD movement are truly a gift to the world. I am so blessed to have been a part of it. Thank you seems so meager compared to the fullness my soul feels. It's really like birth I am so fulfilled to have delivered the baby and yet my soul aches for the pregnancy to continue.

And in 2007

Oh my...BOLD Austin rocked!!! Saturday night was excellent and Sunday was AWESOME!!!!!

All the actresses were spot on for both performances, relaxed, had fun with it, and gave a killer performance...Sunday, during Jillian's moment where she recounts how special the midwife taking her into the shower was, I had tears rolling down my cheeks and my voice was cracking...it was so real for ME and the audience!

We SOLD OUT both shows and (unfortunately) had to turn 10 people away on Saturday...and since Sunday was sold out too we couldn't accommodate them...but they learned that NEXT year they'll just have to buy their tickets earlier than at the door!!

NO media coverage, (which really burns me!) but GREAT audience response and verbal feedback. Had at least a half-dozen people tell me the play and our cast should be on Broadway! LOTS of MEN stopped me afterward to tell me how moving it was!!!! I LOVE THAT!!!

No post partum depression after the performances this year (we did BOLD in 2006 too!)…Just shear fulfillment!!! I spent a good chunk of this morning weeping tears of fulfillment and gratitude.

Wa-HOOOO!!!

- Susan Steffes, BOLD 2007 Organizer, Austin, Texas (yes, Susan was an organizer in 2006 and 2007!)

From BOLD Alaska…

We got special permission to hold our event at The Bear Tooth Theatre and Pub. They had never held a play there before-only movies and live bands. They told us they expected to lose money that night…and we sold out! Actually turned people away (sad) and made money for the theatre-a win-win!

I probably spoke to over 50 people after the show and everyone raved about the play. My husband said it was way better than he expected! The following day I had tons of people coming up to me telling me what a great experience it was.

The most rewarding experience for me was the night of the performance…my entire office showing up, selling out the theatre, and having people come up to me afterwards with tears streaming down their faces, telling me what an amazing play it was.

-Barbara Norton, BOLD 2007 Organizer, Anchorage, Alaska

From BOLD Malta...

The performance was great. It was such a good experience for all of us. The mothers, who acted in the play, were thrilled. They bonded so well together they want to keep on meeting occasionally. They said there's never enough time to talk about their birth experience. It wasn't easy to keep them focused during rehearsals as they kept remembering their own experiences, wanting to talk about it all the time. Believe me, it was the best therapy to come to terms with what they did not like and would like to change.

It was a first experience of performing a play for most of us. Only my sister (Gillian) was a professional actress. The others were all busy mothers, thankful that they could come and have a break from the usual routine, with a difference. They really enjoyed it, saying that it gave them an opportunity to have insights about how they were affected with their own birth experience and how they would make it better, if they could. I am sure that this feeling will be radiated to the people they will be meeting in the future.

We are thinking seriously about combining the play with the official opening of a childbirth education school. The first in Malta.

It felt good to know that we were kind of joined together with other BOLD performances, even though we were separated by the distance.

- Marianne Theuma, BOLD 2006, Malta

In 2006 Marianne was the only childbirth educator in Malta.

From BOLD Houston, Texas...

Whew! - What an experience - we ended up with about 300 people total - our last performance was "standing/sitting on the floor room only" but was very hot - the a/c wasn't very good and it is hot here - but it didn't dampen our enthusiastic cast or audience. The audience was applauding standing up before we were through with the last lines - it was fantastic! We were all so happy.

At our first performance on Friday night we had a crowd of 100 - and they loved it. We had a mother in the audience who cried as she told us that she has totally changed her mind and now can support her daughter who wants to homebirth.

Our second performance on Saturday was really good. Again people were crying and one of the suggestions was to have Kleenex in the audience. We made changes in people's lives obviously.

My organization has been doing the BIRTH Fair in Houston every year for 5 years now and doing outreach talks, etc for several years and this play affected more people than anything we have done to raise the consciousness of our community - we are so very pleased

I am coming down from my high and back to reality now. I had such fun and can't wait until next year - all our actors and in fact everyone who participated is experiencing a high from the event.

- Pat Jones, BOLD 2006, Houston, Texas
  (Pat also produced BOLD 2007 in Houston!)

From BOLD Seattle, Washington in 2006...

OH . . . . MYYY . . .GODDDD! I can hardly believe that we were just getting organized one month ago and didn't have the show cast until August 14!

At the last minute (two weeks ago), we secured our 75-seat venue, thinking "I think we might be able to fill 75 seats." Well we SOLD OUT on Thursday before a blurb was even in the paper. We were getting calls all day Friday from very disappointed people who had waited till the last minute to call. I had my teenagers out front taking names and contact info of people who showed up at the door, so we can contact them for the NEXT performance. My daughter said, "MOM, there are two PREGNANT women waiting here. They REALLY want to see it--Can't we figure out a way to fit them?" We ended up squeezing about 85 people in the space aside from cast and crew!

In 2007, BOLD Organizer Lynn Hughes and her Seattle cast got even BOLDer and organized 11 performances throughout the month of September in the Pudget Sound area. For a woman who has no background in theatre it was quite a producing feat! Lynn writes:

More than 900 people attended one of our many performances of *Birth* or a BOLD Red Tent around Puget Sound!

We definitely got people talking, and we heard at least two stories of pregnant women who came to see the play and, as a result, decided to attempt a VBAC rather than undergo the repeat c/section each had planned. A number of our actors were approached by people on the street or at social gatherings, recognizing them as a member of the *Birth* cast and telling them how much they enjoyed the show! We got some momentum going, and we hope to bring *Birth* to more audiences in the future (we are talking to one middle school teacher and a Seattle alternative High School who are interested in bringing *Birth* to their schools).

One of the most exciting aspects of Puget Sound BOLD was the community support. Seattle author and childbirth guru, Penny Simkin sparkled in the role of Amanda for our Gala Opening Night at Edmonds. What a thrill for everyone! Penny wrote to members of the production the next day,

"My routine seems a little mundane after the past couple of weeks and especially, after last night. What a thrill! Thanks to you for giving me a taste of the "acting life," but mostly for your kindness and support to me and your moving performances last night. I deeply appreciate that all of you are helping to open the eyes of the public to the fact that the birth day is not "just another day in a woman's life." How a woman gives birth matters -- deeply and permanently -- to her, her child and to her family. She remembers the experience for all her life -- not only what happened, but also how she felt and how she was cared for. You illustrate that perfectly as you enact the stories. Your efforts will help your audiences make choices that will provide them with the care that they want and deserve, and that will result in more fulfilling memories of their births."

\- Lynn Hughes, BOLD 2007 Organizer,
Pudget Sound, Washington

From BOLD Montana...

WE DID IT! The cast and audience had a great time and were very, very excited about the play. Some women from the cast and audience have indicated that they would like to do it again next year - could there be a more positive statement?

I spent many many hours publicizing and promoting BOLD in the community. I applied for and received donated ad space in the local paper; I copied 50 posters and had two moms help me put them up all over town; I mailed a personal invitation to all the OB's and Family Doctors who deliver at our local Hospital, as well as to the local midwives offering home birth services, not only inviting them to come to attend the BOLD performance but also asking them to sit on a panel for the public talkback that was scheduled to follow the reading of the play. To my great disappointment, not a single maternity care provider attended the play let alone offered to sit on the talkback panel. After all the publicity I did our turnout was 20-30 people, actually not bad for our conservative community, but still I would have liked to see at least two or three times as many people.

We hope BOLD will take roots and grow in Montana. The climate in this Northern mountain state is such that it may take a while and the seedling will need lots of tending, but if anything we are a tenacious people and will patiently wait for the seasons to change.

> - Marianne Donch, BOLD 2006 Organizer,
> Bozeman, Montana

From BOLD Washington, DC…

Our reading of *Birth* was a victim of a bit of a weather situation. A hurricane was predicted to hit Washington DC on the night of our show. With limited advanced ticket sales, a venue without parking, and lights out in most residential neighborhoods near us, it seemed our event just wasn't going to happen the way we hoped, but something happened shortly before curtain time. No, the clouds didn't clear, in fact, the winds kicked up and the rain poured down; but that didn't stop the crowds. We played to a standing room only crowd, exceeded our fundraising goals, and made a significant contribution to discussions about how to make maternity care in Washington DC mother-friendly. Our show was a success in the worst of weather conditions because people not only want to see *Birth*, they NEED to see it. They need a safe forum to tell the truth about their birth experience, to educate themselves or loved ones about the state of birth today, and to feel empowered to take action to make the world better for birthing moms.

I think the power of BOLD is its ability to touch communities at this micro-level. BOLD has the ability to change lives of mothers and their families community by community through the transformative properties of theatre.

- Angela Lauria, Director, BOLD 2006, Washington DC (and BOLD 2006 Coordinator!)

From BOLD Memphis...

Women came with their young daughters and college students came to see the show for a class that they were taking. From their comments and their reaction papers they learned a lot about birth that will inform the choices that they make when they decide to have children of their own. A major breakthrough for the students was to see women depicting birth in other positions besides on their backs. Their papers also addressed the fact that the emotions of the women and how they were treated during the births helped to illustrate why knowledge, access and choices need to get better in our community.

An audience member said that she really appreciated seeing the journey of Jillian's character, especially the communication that birth can be ecstatic for a woman. It was noted on more than one occasion that Jillian's transformation helps women see that birth and attitudes about birth can be changed.

As a result of the show an online Yahoo group of Memphis Moms called Alternamamas had a follow-up discussion and potluck to further talks about the play and the Memphis birthing scene. The midwives on the Talkback Panel also brought in the Ricki Lake documentary The Business of Being Born and featured the directors of Birth on their panel. The director of Birth is working on a hosting a series prenatal information sessions with a doula and a childbirth educator that are going to be free and open to the public at a local wellness facility.

A local ob contacted the directors of Birth to let them know that one of her patients was able to do a VBAC after seeing the show and switching providers.

Most rewarding: Seeing people without stage experience pull off strong performances and knowing that what we were doing was going to help change the birth scene in Memphis!

-       Kimberly Baker, BOLD 2007 Organizer,
Memphis, Tennessee

From BOLD Toledo, Ohio…

I loaded up the car the night before our performance after 2 days of tech rehearsals...then at the theater setting up at 8:30am. Dress rehearsal from 9-12. We had a nice relaxing lunch at a tea shop, with pictures and stories and we were all back at the theater by five. Our director was up the whole night before and also the afternoon working on a slide program to project on the screen behind the actors. 5-6pm was the last minute rehearsal, with me running around setting up ticket sales table, and other last minute tasks. 6:30pm people started coming, doors opened and the excitement was intoxicating. My music cue did not work but I finally went out and did my welcome speech. (I was very nervous But when it was for real in front of an audience...I came through!)

Then it started, one story after another going VERY well. No major mistakes, some lighting problems, but great overall. During intermission I could tell everyone was enjoying it. We were all interviewed by a local television station. The second act was even better! Jillian made us laugh, Natalie and Sandy made us cry. The cast got a standing ovation and the audience response was very positive.

Everyone I spoke to after the performance said the play was riveting, truthful, well-written and very much needed in our community. We also had the "real" Jillian and her whole family who had never seen the play before. I am already thinking about next year and things I would change. Am I crazy??

A friend gave me a magnet that said, "Think big, if that doesn't work, THINK BIGGER!" So BOLD women, Think bigger for next year!

- Carolyn Self, BOLD 2007 Organizer, Toledo, Ohio

From BOLD Fresno, California...

Wow... where to start?? What a wonderful group of women we put together! Let me first say that myself and Chanah are very active Birth professionals, and had more than a few deliveries during the whole process, in fact one of Chanah's clients delivered after the Fri night performance and she made it back for the Sat one!! In our cast Dawn, Melissa,Gena and Cheryl all have babies. Most of our rehearsals took place amid crawlers, nurslings and crying, and we wouldn't have traded a minute of it!! GJ and Stacey are old theatre buffs and stated at the end of our performances that they have NEVER had such a wonderful time!

As for the performances; Friday, the morning of opening night, was our first time actually on the stage. Friday night we tried to relax before the performance, we were all getting pretty nervous. Gena and I drank a glass of wine! I was worried we would have a very small audience.. we did comp - we gave many of the tickets to young women either pregnant or thinking about it in the near future. We were surprised to find a decent audience (for Fresno!). The audience was very positive and laughed, and at times cried. Act two I think we felt more relaxed (or this could be my assumption, clouded by the second glass of wine I drank during intermission, anyway, I was more relaxed!).GJ's part, the character Natalie, brought a silence that you could cut to the audience, a few women were reliving some painful memories. Gena played the character Lisa and there was not a dry eye in the audience. Fresno has a 37% c-section rate, so many women could relate, and many members of the International Cesarean Awareness Network were there. The character Janet's birth was very special for the actor Dawn who played her, as her twins were born via c-section (and she thanks Karen deeply for giving her the birth she wanted!!).

- Lisa Gartin, BOLD 2007 Organizer, Fresno, California

From BOLD Denver, Colorado...

Opening night was a surprise as we only sold about 23 tickets in advance and ended up having about 90 people come to a 100 seat venue. The next Friday night was a sell out and we had to turn people away at the door because we were out of room. The performances went great and we got rave reviews from our audiences. One of our actors has a dad who's an OB and after the play he had a lengthy conversation with our actress who played Sandy. He said that he views himself as the advocate for the baby and gets really frustrated when the moms he works with are reluctant to consent to a c-section when he feels one is necessary. He said that seeing Sandy's story reminded him that the experience isn't ALL about the baby, but mom's process as well and that he could do better to take a few moments to check in with mom and see how she is feeling and just to take a moment to hear the mom side and listen to her and create a space where the mom is involved in the decision and not just him as the OB. He said it was a great play and I could hear him laughing behind me during the performance.

Another great story is that of another of our actors, Anita. She played Jillian and has a 19 year old son. He came to opening night and she told us that after the play she had a great discussion with him and he was pretty much brought to tears to see the stories and the way birth is treated sometimes. It was quite moving to hear that a young man who isn't married, doesn't have any kids could relate to a play about women giving birth. I think he will be a great advocate for his future wife and baby.

I think the most rewarding part of the BOLD experience was on opening night when the actors and stage mangers and I were warming up before the performance. We were all standing in a circle facing each other and I felt this overwhelming feeling of gratitude and love for these women who had sacrificed their free time, and put their families on wacky schedules in order to help me put together something that I feel so passionate about. I can truly say that I love all of the women that were a part of this and I am so thankful for all of their help and talents.

- Miranda Cacek, BOLD 2007 Organizer, Denver, Colorado

From BOLD Chicago...

Alright, let's review this weekend! We had 3 performances - - Friday, Saturday, and Sunday. I was very calm on Friday, everything was done, and ready to go. My husband came home from work early, brought me lunch, and helped me to prepare all the materials. He had stayed up late the night before helping to fold all the programs and working on the Talkback sheet.

My in-laws arrive to babysit and Pete and I leave in separate cars to go to the theater so I was free to play my Dixie Chicks CD as loudly as I wanted to get psyched for the play. We used the song, "Lullaby," as our last song after Jillian's birth.

Of course, by the time I arrived at the theater, I was already feeling a little weepy and jittery. Just as I pull into the parking space, next to one of the co-directors, Karin, and open my car door to get out, my cell phone rings. I pick it up and my friend and ICAN (International Cesarean Awareness Network) of Chicago board member, Liz, is calling. She's supposed to be picking up roses for the actresses and meeting me at the theater so I assume she's calling me about some last minute details. Instead, she says, "I had the baby. I had the baby. I had the baby!" I am so stunned I cannot comprehend what she says. "What? The baby? What do you mean you had the baby?" She was not due until the first week of October – almost a month away. Eventually I begin to understand and comprehend what she's saying. In the meantime, Karin is standing there wondering why the heck I don't get out of my car and get in the theater so we can get started with setting up. At that point, I really do begin to cry, and scream all at once. She had the baby, she had the baby! And it was a VBAC (vaginal birth after cesarean)! A 3 hour labor! And here she was telling me she had the baby and then she told me that she had already arranged for someone else to go get the flowers for the actresses! Isn't that hilarious! What a way to start the night! Of course, I saw several other ICAN members that night, and we were so excited for Liz and

151

for BIRTH! I told all the cast members at the Blessingway about Liz, and then we had groaning cake, and I gave each actress and director a red stone to hold on to or to put in their pocket as they told their birth stories on stage. And, yes, one stone did drop in the middle of a scene and go rolling across the stage! It was just the perfect beginning to a really meaningful, enlightening weekend.

Lastly, I learned some more things about my own births this weekend, and I decided to take a cue from Jillian and ask if I can attend some other people's births -- why not?

- Julie Lambert, BOLD 2007 Organizer, Chicago, Illinois

From BOLD Lawrence, Kansas...

Hello all BOLD women,

Here, in Lawrence, Kansas, we just did 2 shows at our Lawrence Arts Center. I am just writing now because I have been completely overwhelmed with the acting thing (I was Jillian) and trying to pull this off and mothering (mother of 3 homeschooled children) and attending births (I am a homebirth midwife) and organizing. But we did it, we really, really did it.

Our rehearsals were full of mamas and nursing babies and toddlers and a very lovely rapt 9 year old girl helping to entertain those wee ones. I am a midwife and felt the desperate need to stretch myself beyond my "one mama, one baby, one family at a time" vision, and just throw myself into this global action. As Jillian, I have learned so so much. And witnessing the intimate personal struggles of each cast member, I have learned so much.

My goodness.

Thank you, Karen, for providing this avenue of dialogue in our community. We so needed it. I cannot begin to explain, in an email, what I have experienced, nor what the beautiful courageous BOLD women I have been working with have experienced. My heart is full and bursting and tired. Thank you, thank you, thank you.

On behalf of our Lawrence BOLD members and our Lawrence, Kansas community, I thank you.

I am hoping next year will be much easier!

Off to bed, without rehearsing my lines....

- Brenda Frankenfeld, BOLD 2007 Organizer, Lawrence, Kansas

From BOLD Ontario, Canada...

Okay... so it's show time... we have 3.5 hours to show time and all is calm and relaxed. The set is up, the actresses blessed and ready to roll, the panelists are ready and we have fourteen seats left for people who walk in without a ticket in hand. We have had great publicity and promotion and a very supportive community about raising awareness. Our info tables are packed and we have CIMS and Baby Friendly material being handed out with the programmes and some people have indicated that they want to do it again next year.

So.... as the producer, shouldn't I be more nervous.... am I missing something??

> \- Melissa Cowl, BOLD 2007 Organizer, Alliston, Ontario, Canada

From BOLD Northhampton, Massachusetts...

There is still a tremendous amount of buzz about the BOLD events. Many have commented how moving and provocative the production was. Women enjoyed sharing their birth experiences and thinking about the changes they would like to see in maternity care.

The most rewarding experience for me was selling out the performances, watching our cast create a community of friends, drinking champagne at the post-show party, watching the ripple effect of women feeling empowered by having witnessed the play and moving forward with taking control of their own health care choices. What an experience!

> \- Kristin Lane, BOLD 2007 Organizer, Northampton, Massachusetts

From BOLD New York City...

The performances were great – our innovative professional director, Heidi Miami Marshall, used a lot of multi-media techniques with the actors speaking into video cameras at times which made the experience rich and fast-paced. The actors were all professional New York City actors - challenging as I was walking into a completely new experience for me and the other midwives producing the show and we were all trying to make the play all that it could be.

It was clear who was in the audience by the different parts of *Birth* that received laughs. The moments like, "You pooped." caused much laughter from the entire audience but the descriptions of the crunchy granola midwife and such sent the midwives who attended into hysterics.

I think an important point that the play makes is that working with a person with the designation of "midwife" "ob" "nurse" or even "doula" does not guarantee a particular experience but that you have a right to find someone with whom you are comfortable sharing this much-more-than-just-one-day experience.

- Hilary Prager, BOLD 2007 Organizer, New York City

From BOLD Wilmington, North Carolina...

So many wonderful memories from working on this play!

Our cast was made up of five professional actresses and three birth professionals (one CPM, one doula, one apprenticing CPM); broken down another way - four mommies, four non-mommies. Everyone was learning from everyone else about acting and about childbirth.

Opening night was absolutely electric! I cried, and I'd seen the play many, many times before.! The run of the show went way too quickly.

- Kristi Kretzter, BOLD 2007 Organizer, Wilmington, North Carolina

From BOLD Asheville, North Carolina...

Here's how we did a blessingway with our cast before our
performances:

The woman leading it began by making a short pathway for each
actor to walk into the space. She lit 7 day novena candles (tall
candles in glass jars) to have each woman walk through. When
we got into her circle, she had laid our an altar with a childbirth
education pelvis, cloth uterus and baby on it. In the middle was a
bowl with a bead for each woman. She asked us to call in anyone
we wished to be with us. Most actors called in their grandmothers
who had passed. At the end she asked us to thank them for being
with us and to release them. This may be too pagan for your
group, but ours was fine with it. She asked each actor to state what
they were feeling at that moment. We heard, excited, tired, and a
few other feelings.

I would suggest reading this quote from our program:
There's an African story of birth where the women gather and
send you across the river, and as you walk across this log across
the river you head out with these women. As you go across the
narrowest part you're alone. No one can be there with you, and
as you emerge onto the other side of the river, all the women who
have ever given birth are there to meet you. (Liz Koch, as quoted
in Mothering the New Mother).

I would bless everyone by saying something like: A blessingway
is often done in lieu of a baby shower to mark the transition
from pregnancy to motherhood. Each of you has labored in your

preparation for this show. You are now in transition, preparing to push as you give birth to your characters on stage. As you become your characters, you are honoring not only the women whose stories you tell, but every woman who has made the journey into motherhood. May you be blessed and know that the work you are doing is important to your community and the larger community of motherhood. May you find within you the spirit of your grandmothers as you do this important work. Have no fear. The baby is at the door. Have no fear. Your time has come. Have no fear. You are giving life to your characters. May you do so with courage. Your work is a gift. You are blessed. Be BOLD.

The woman who blessed us placed one hand on our belly and the other on our foreheads. As she blessed each of us, she had each who had been blessed go behind her blessing each cast member so that by the end of the circle we had all been blessed by the woman who led us and by each of our fellow actors. Some of them laid hands on different parts of the body - our mouths so that the words that fell from them would be what the audience needed to hear, etc. Some of us just hugged each other.

Then she released the circle and we told each other to break a leg. We all filed out through the candle pathway. Candles were extinguished and the stage set for the curtain to rise.

- Desire O'Clair, BOLD 2006 Organizer, Asheville, North Carolina

BOLD talkbacks

"I want to know why women want a prada bag, but they are not interested in tuning in to this core power that's available for them giving birth?"

- Dr. Christiane Northrup, author of *Mother-Daughter Wisdom, The Wisdom of Menopause* and *Women's Bodies, Women's Wisdom* , BOLD 2006, New York City

The first night our talkback that night was far greater then we could have dreamed, we had 50 people stay and had to kick them out at 12am!!! A pediatrician was in the audience, asked if he could come up and join the panel, then at the end, asked for permission to join us for the Saturdays panel!!

Saturday night we had the panel introduce themselves and opened up the microphone for questions. Many MEN came up with questions. The question of choices made because of fear of litigation was brought up by a Lawyer…whose wife was very pregnant…!! Our OB answered very truthfully for both sides, very balanced. The topic of water birth came up, it does happen in Fresno, at home… and we discussed how to bring it in to the hospital! Informed choice and consent came up both nights… women and men know that this is NOT happening as it should, especially with VBAC (vaginal birth after cesarean). The audience both nights had to eventually take it "outside" as we were WAY over our time for the theatre!!!!

- BOLD 2007, Fresno, California

One thing all of you can do today, right now, is go to your local media and say: where were you today? Where were you on a Sunday when a sold-out play was taking place in your community about one of the most important things on earth: birth? Hold the media accountable!

- Kitty Ernst Young, BOLD 2007,
Santa Rosa, California

One highlight was speaking to people in the audience and finding out what they thought about birth and "interviewing" them about their thoughts on birth and what their peers think about it. I spoke to a handful of college students and some of the women said that they did not talk about birth and were learned a great deal. The young men I spoke to were surprised to hear that birth was so meaningful to women, they had thought of birth as a medical procedure and had not thought much about the emotional component. I asked them what they would tell their wives (in future years) and they said that they would tell them to get educated and find out more information. It made me think, we always talk about educating the women but if men were behind the cause it might change faster. Men have a great deal of power in this country. Maybe we should focus on teaching the men more intently and at a young age?

A professor from Boston University asked a very interesting question at the BOLD Talkback. She had brought a bunch of her students to watch the play and she said that the topic of "birth" is not part of her women's studies curriculum. She said that it is quite telling that if birth is not considered a women's studies issue that we have a great deal of education to cover. The Talkbacks also covered the issues of malpractice insurance costing so much, which puts pressure for c-sections, What can people do to make changes to improve maternity care? Write letters and tell their stories!

-    BOLD 2007, Boston, Massachusetts

At our BOLD Talkbacks women stood up and made it clear that this area WANTS AND NEEDS midwives, options, choices, etc. Our only birth center is in the process of closing, we want women, we want water births, we want doctors who will listen, who will measure success by more than apgar scores. It was a good dialogue. It was great to see the responses of the audience. Many women, pregnant, new mothers, grandmothers, you name it. All praising this show... how wonderful it is.

The next night a woman asked the Talkback panel for their response to the play - if they felt like seeing it from a woman's perspective would change the way they practiced.

One OB dominated the discussion - saying he felt like this was first and foremost entertainment - (to which a woman quickly piped up and reminded him these are TRUE stories). He said he didn't feel it was representative of this area (to which women stood up and said "Um, hello - THIS IS!!!"). He said if he was THAT out of the loop, and there was that kind of feelings, then he wasn't doing his job, none of them were doing their job and they needed to retire then and there. He started saying something (hate to try to quote verbatim) basically saying that he would know if this was going on here, and that he didn't feel like it was. Women stood up and said it was. Another point made was "How can women let you know that this was their experience? They can't very well waltz in and say "hey you suck!" The OB responded that they have 6 week postpartum checkups & they usually ask how things are going - ask the dad how the mom is doing, etc. It was pointed out by several women that at 6 weeks postpartum you're barely brushing your teeth much less processing your birth!!! That for so many women its months, if not YEARS later, that they talk to other women and find out "OMG - that wasn't how it HAD TO BE! There are other choices? options? you mean, my doctor didn't tell me I didn't HAVE to x,y,z?! I feel betrayed!"

I pointed out that cast members, local women, played parts that mocked their own birth. The character I played, Natalie - her birth WAS my first birth! He turned the light back to me - asking WHAT I did to recover, what I did to take responsibility back - I responded "I HAD A HOMEBIRTH!"

He & the other OB did discuss ways to let providers know - that they did want to know - even if one letter alone didn't change the way they did business, that over time, if they saw it was a pattern they may rethink how they treat women. They talked about how they practice defensive medicine, that they're not going to risk losing everything they have worked so hard for a woman to have a satisfying birth experience.

Finally - the most awesome part of it all. The director stood up and told the panelist about how women NEED to be heard, that these women are dealing with the messes they leave behind when they go home to their families without a worry, that she only hopes they have the balls they claim to - about the importance of birth & how many women are so traumatized, hurt, dejected, sad about what should be the most beautiful day of their lives and how a simple nice gesture can go a long ways, how body language can make a big difference - she used the Fuck word a time or two - appropriately I might add lol... (The balls reference was about the OB saying had never have the balls to give birth himself – he's so glad not to be a woman).

She got a standing ovation and the biggest round of applause and whistling the whole auditorium had ever seen!!!! And she ended it with "And I hope the next time you care for a woman, you remember the words of these women!!"

- BOLD 2007, Pensacola, Florida

We had such amazing members of our BOLD Talkback panel. We had midwives, doulas, obs, activists, authors, women representing marginalized populations such as the lesbian community and incarcerated women, nurses. We discussed what birth in New York today is like. That led to what options women have, what could/should be changed, how to trust your provider in a moment of "crisis", transparency in the health care system. Our OBs were all men and they were wonderful. At one BOLD Talkback the OB on our panel started off by thanking the playwright and founder of BOLD, Karen Brody (who was in the audience!) for writing a play that – in his opinion – told the truth about childbirth today.

- BOLD 2007, New York City

I think it's important to note that since the talkback some fathers have approached me to ask why they are so often left out of all of this. They noted that they often feel left out and intimidated by the birthing community - the "sorority" as one called it. I didn't think we had done that in our talkback - we actually talked a lot about how important the couple is, how much stronger they are when they are both educated in the process of birth and possible interventions etc, but these two dads noted that they felt unsure of their place in birth. Something else to think about...how do we include fathers in birth?

- BOLD 2007, Flagstaff, Arizona

We published stats in our playbill along with some really pertinent information - we had cesarean rates for every local hospital in a 4 county area - HOSPITAL BY HOSPITAL! It was great. Our high risk hospital had a LOWER cesarean rate than the one that is in my own town - what is considered by far the worst (aka "hack & slash, Inc.").

So at the talkback I come to find out the OB on our Talkback panel only arrived in about the last 15 minutes of the play. She didn't even really see the play, which bummed me out. She's the head doctor at a new hospital in the area - a sister hospital of the high risk hospital two counties over which has a great reputation for being on the more mother-friendly side. We had really high hopes needless to say. So you can imagine my disappointment when she answered a question about empowering women with how she didn't understand women who said they felt like a "failure" - she kept saying "If the baby is healthy & the mom is ok - why would you feel like a failure - if everyone's healthy then the birth was a success."

Ah yes, thank you for reminding me WHY WE HAD THE PLAY IN THE FIRST PLACE!!!

Now, mind you - we had provided her with information on what the play was about, and the principles BOLD stood for... she was so pro-woman when she talked to my talk back coordinator. But where the HELL did this come from!? I shook my head, then stood up and told her, I wished she'd have seen the play - that really - women feel like failures not ONLY because their birth outcome wasn't as planned but also when their power & voice is taken away. That women who have doctors and nurses and everyone BUT THEM making the decision and when the baby is DELIVERED FROM THEM and birth is something that happens TO THEM, *THAT'S* when you feel like a failure. That's what makes it such a huge sadness. There is no sense of accomplishment. Drugs, machines, doctors, medicines, pills – all of these things do the work. They make you have contractions, THEY break your water, THEY make you dilate, THEY HELP YOU push, THEY THEY THEY - where are WE in the picture?! WE are the mothers, WE are the voice that needs to be heard, WE NEED TO KNOW and LET OTHER WOMEN KNOW that WE CAN DO THIS!!! That we don't NEED those things. How many women walk out of their birth with healthy babies, healthy themselves, the end result was what they wanted, but they feel powerless, they are totally disconnected – they're just the incubator, they bring the baby to the hospital, and take the baby home, and they're no part of the in between!

Sigh.

- BOLD 2007 Pensacola, Florida

BOLD men speak

Peace and blessings to you Karen Brody. Thank you so much for
such a lovely monologue. As a father of four and a grandfather of
11, I was not aware of some of the challenges that some women
go through. I am aware that you have seen your play done several
times, I must say that I don't believe you've seen it performed like
how we did it in Maui. No script in hand, just full theater, I would
say at its best. It would be nice if you could come to see this.
My desire is that more men would come out to see this blessed
production. Robin has been a chosen blessing that has brought
together such a cast to present this wonderful gift. We feel as
though this presentation has been ordained by energy source and
after watching its effect after the first show we now know so. Give
thanks for allowing yourself to be a medium for this gift. We hope
to see you. May spirit continue to guide.

Peace and Blessings,

>   - Baba Kauna, theater coach, Maui, Hawaii,
>   BOLD 2007

Karen,

Though we've never met or spoken, I feel like I've got to know
you over the past few months through your correspondences with
the BOLD Organizer here in Asheville. I've been reflecting on

our experience with the play. For myself, I know the journey was enlightening. I don't feel like an expert, but I certainly know more about birth than I did before and feel comfortable holding the conversation.

I feel like BOLD could very well redefine Labor Day, much in the way the Vagina Monologues has taken over V-Day.

Unless you haven't heard, BOLD was a huge success in Asheville. I haven't received exact figures yet, but I feel like we were very close to setting a box office record for attendance at a CATALYST series (non-main stage) show at North Carolina Stage Company.

- Josh Batenhorst
Director, Asheville, North Carolina, BOLD 2006

I went through two births with my wife, it was so strange and kind of disappointing that I felt so helpless, I couldn't do anything. I realize now that it should be all about her and her doing it and the last thing that anyone needs while they are concentrating during labor is to worry about what someone else is up to. I finally get it.

- Audience member and professor, BOLD 2006,
Lynchburg, Virginia

BOLD ripples

Dear Midwives, Doulas, Lactation Educators, Nurses, OB experts,

We at Kaiser have been looking at ways to make both our care in the clinic, and our care at Maui Memorial, more responsive to mother and baby's needs. The play, "Birth", was another spark, in keeping this dialogue and hope alive. "Dr. B" is inviting you, (and some others, who don't have email) to meet at her home on October 14 from 12 noon to 3 pm. "Dr. R" also plans to be there-to listen to your input, on ways to make care to women, better. This would include how best to facilitate transfers from home births, and ways to make the hospital more "homelike" and supportive for mothers and babies. We hope we'll be able to have future meetings, and thought this would be a start.

Let's have a nurturing, beautiful potluck together.

- Carol Thomason, Nurse-Midwife/Lactation Consultant, Maui, Hawaii

I wanted to share with all of you something that I shared at rehearsal tonight about the power of this play. I just did a six-week postpartum visit today with a young woman whom I worked with. She is in her early twenties, a survivor of numerous deep wounds from her childhood, including family suicide, sexual abuse and assault. She is now married to a man she loves and when we sat together, she said, " I had a wonderful birth, a home birth, and I

167

am proud of myself!" It was absolutely true and she was holding her healthy, chubby, breastfed baby as she said it. She was sharing a profound life change for her. For me, I felt that all we have done with our organization Birthnet over the 8 years we have been doing it was just validated because this young woman came to her decisions about her birth and her baby because, as a student about 5 or 6 years ago, she was in one of the classes at SUNY Albany where we came and talked about choices for women when they are birthing and showed a film about options and choices.. It galvanized her to arrive where she is today. Sooooo, I see this play in the same light. If you think about it, with a local surgical birth rate of over 33%, if 300 women see this play over the two shows, 100 or more of those women who have had children will have had surgery and this play may be speaking to them and helping them heal. And/or 100 of those women are headed towards a surgical birth or other intervention, possibly unnecessary, and they may learn something from this play that will help them make other choices. Think about the power of that! Even if we reach just one or two of those, and frankly, we already have with our actors, we are changing the future for these women and their families. So, I know everyone is busy and everything may be piling up in your life, but all the work for this production is so IMPORTANT and vital and you are making it happen for each of those women who need to celebrate or heal or learn new options, as well as yourselves, I hope. So, thank you for all you are doing and keep on keepin on.

- Betsy Mercogliano, birth activist, an extra in the play, birth coach, and one of the producers /organizers of BOLD 2007 in Troy, New York

I played Beth in the Chicago production of BIRTH. The most rewarding aspect of the experience for me was hearing my cast mates say how much they had learned about childbirth from having been involved in the play. Henci Goer called BIRTH "a powerful new means of communicating the importance of birth issues to the public." And she is absolutely right. Events such as a BIRTH performance allow us to reach a new audience, rather than just 'preaching to the choir'.

On a more personal note, I want to share something that had an even more profound impact on me. I had the opportunity to meet you, Karen, this past spring when you came to Chicago for the staged reading of BIRTH and a kind of a talkback panel at Sweet Pea yoga studio the next day. I was telling everyone about how my daughter's birth was the single most traumatic experience of my life, and that afterwards all I heard from my friends and family was that having a healthy baby was all that mattered. Although I am aghast to admit that I can't remember exactly what you said, you asked me something like, if everyone is telling me that a healthy baby is all that matters, how did I know that it wasn't true? That made me think. I remember saying something like, "Oh, I don't know, I guess just something inside of me knew it was wrong." that moment was a kind of epiphany for me, like "MY MIND ROCKS!" :) I know it might sound silly, but what you said to me that day has really stayed with me. And having been involved in the production of BIRTH has allowed me to finally make peace with my daughter's birth as well. Were it not for my traumatic experience, I never would have met any of my 'BIRTH sisters' and friends from my ICAN (International Cesarean Awareness Network) and Homebirth Meetups. So I guess what I'm trying to say to BOLD is I don't think you have to worry about not doing enough.

I'll leave you with one of my favorite poems:

If I can stop one heart from breaking,
I shall not live in vain;
If I can ease one life the aching,
Or cool one pain,
Or help one fainting robin
Unto his nest again,
I shall not live in vain.

~Emily Dickinson

-    Bold Chicago cast member, 2007

We are already making a difference for families here in Northern Arizona. Our BOLD performance inspired a group of labor and delivery nurses at the hospital to bring "The Business of Being Born" to Flagstaff this month. Our talkback started not only the discussion about the need for a birth network to happen here - but the actual formation of it! We've applied to be a charter of the Arizona Birth Network and our community is coming together to help get the word out to women about what is available to them to have the best birth experience possible.

-    Flagstaff, Arizona. BOLD 2007

BOLD birth stories

Many people ask me why I am volunteering so many hours of my time to bring the play BIRTH to the world this Labor Day. My story is a simple one of karma - giving back to the universe for the last minute miracle of an empowered (though imperfect) birth. I gave birth about 12 weeks ago with a lot of help from my incredible, amazing, life-changing doula who I met when I was 38 weeks pregnant. At 36 weeks my OB started talking about a scheduled C based on the baby's size which at the time according to the ultrasound looked to be 8 lbs and they were estimating the famous 10 lb baby which I'd *never* be able to push out (according to the OB that is!). I'm sure you know this drill.

Completely uneducated about birth beyond "What to Expect When You're Expecting," and the one-day class offered by the hospital, the idea of a scheduled C sounded okay to me - but I was still a bit confused and wanted to ask around before I made a decision. My questioning online led me to a conversation with a doula and another with a midwife who opened up my eyes to so much I had no idea was going on around me.

In 3 weeks, I sucked up all the info my doula could offer and prepared myself for a drug free delivery. But it wasn't meant to be. In the end - after 2 hours of pushing with the baby's heart rate dropping - I did have an emergency c-section. But with my doula's help I feel comfortable I did all I could do to avoid one (though I know I was still pushed into it faster than I would have been if I were working with a better OB team). After I had the baby I really wanted to do something to help mainstream mamas like me get exposure to the concept that childbirth is a natural process and not a medical one.

For me, having no exposure to a non-medicalized model of pregnancy, I viewed anything outside the "What to Expect" model as "squatting in the rice patty - certain death for mom and baby." I had no idea women's bodies were so amazing. Even though I had a c, I was able to experience my body working and it was amazing. As each contraction rolled through and the 'pain' seemed so overwhelming I felt not just connected to other mothers - but to the entire planet... was this how the ocean felt the day of the tsunami? It was awesome to see myself stretch literally, figurative, and emotionally in way I never knew possible. (Have I mentioned how amazing my doula was - she got me so far in our 3 weeks together).

One of the things I think is so powerful about this play is that it takes a non-judgmental stance - it tells the stories - COMMON STORIES - of women giving birth today. It says let's take an honest look at what's going on with birth in America (the west?) and let's start to talk about it. Is this what we really want? Is this what we deserve?

All productions of Birth On Labor Day (BOLD) are to be followed by what we call a BOLD talk back where these issues are discussed. I think this offers an opening for someone who maybe made the decision to schedule a cesarean (like I might have) to release some of their "birth baggage" and maybe even get themselves emotionally in a place where they could have a VBAC (vaginal birth after cesarean) or even heck a HBAC (home birth after cesarean)!

That's what the BOLD movement is about - not just patting people in the birth community on the back, not just supporting women who are already see birth as a natural process, but finding ways to open the dialogue through the noise of the medical community, the Discovery Channel, the What to Expect/Girlfriend's Guides, and to reach out to women who otherwise wouldn't be open to the idea that birth is actually a natural process that our bodies were specifically designed to participate in.

As a busy first time mom, with a new baby and a new job, it's hard to find time to help make BOLD a reality - I'm sure you all have conflicts that make this hard for you in your own ways - but if we don't do this who will? The pharmaceutical companies and insurance companies have millions set aside to spread their propaganda. We need to BEBOLD and raise our voices loudly so we too can be heard!

- Angela Lauria, BOLD 2006 Coordinator

I'll start with how I came to BOLD and then get into my birth stories…

The play was performed in Austin last year but I didn't get to see it. This spring I saw the 'ad' for BOLD on my doula list and knew it was something I wanted to be a part of. I didn't dream I'd be the one organizing it. With no one else from my area organizing it (at least not at that point) I realized I couldn't let BIRTH go unseen…so here I am! As a birth doula my goal is to provide education, encouragement, empowerment and support. Knowing the facts is only one part of decision making but it's a part that is so often left out in medicalized maternal care. Women are led to trust their doctors without questioning…that's crazy! Knowledge and informed consent are what every woman deserves, what every woman needs, to have an empowered birth. BOLD let's women see for themselves the consequences of uninformed and unempowered birth…though non-judgmental in its delivery it is hard to come away from BIRTH without feeling those women deserved more. BRAVO Karen and THANK YOU Angela.

My birth stories…

I have 3 boys: the first was a premature SROM without contractions and since I hadn't had a Group B Strep test done the doc was worried about infection…my doula was out of state and although she tried to help me ask the right questions (via the phone) I felt pretty scared and vulnerable and so agreed to the induction (after a few hours of walking the halls to try and get contractions going). It was horrible! I lasted 7 hours without any pain meds and then when my RN told me she had to leave me for a c-section. I freaked out…I NEEDED a woman present or I wasn't going to be able to cope…so at 5 cm I got the epidural…the anesthesiologist hit a nerve and I darn near flew off the table…followed by my heart rate and respiration dropping to where I was put on oxygen and I thought I was going to die because I couldn't move anything, even my eyes (outer body experience). Well, they finally got everything leveled out and I went on to push out my baby boy…who had trouble nursing for 8 weeks but we kept at it and didn't supplement (other than expressed breast milk from a supplemental nursing system and a cup). My first RN was wonderfully supportive but the RN that replaced her when she had to leave was a drill sergeant and mean. My doctor was supportive but I think overly reactive…I don't think I needed to be induced…at least not so quickly. Labor from the time of induction was 8 hours. They took my son (after initial contact and breastfeeding) for 2 hours (my husband was with him). The ancients visited me in my room that night and held me close (it still makes me cry to think on that moment). I mourned this birth. And so I became a doula…to provide for other women what I didn't have and felt I needed…a woman there for me offering information, constant emotional support and encouragement.

Baby # 2 I was put on bed rest for premature labor but I was let up at 37 weeks and he stayed put until 41+ weeks. Again I had SROM without contractions but this time it was different. Doulas #1 and #2 were present and it was wonderful. After 4 hours and no contractions the doctor suggested that since I had a slow leak that he "finish it off" by tearing a larger hole in the sac…I agreed. Labor was 4 glorious hours of walking and swaying, listening to music, smelling essential oils and a lot of moaning. I wanted to labor naked and even though this made the nurses uncomfortable (heaven knows why - it felt right to me). He was posterior but turned before birth. When our baby boy was born he never left our side. In retrospect I wish I would have labored more at home, but all in all it was a good birth. I felt empowered, supported and proud. I rejoiced in this birth.

Baby 3 was born at 41+ weeks as well. Doula #3 was present. This time labor started as cramping and progressed to stronger contractions. When I got to the hospital I was 6cm and 90% effaced. I still wish I would have stayed home longer but I was nervous he would come quickly and I didn't want to deliver in the car during the 20 minute ride. I actually wanted to have a home birth but that freaked my husband out too much and the birthing center wasn't a good match for us. Regardless of the hospital setting, baby #3 had a wonderful entry…I walked, I kneeled, I sang, I moaned and I cursed. I refused the hep-lock and once in final phase of active labor. I refused additional monitoring. Labor was 12 long hard hours. I really came into my power with this birth.

> - Susan Steffes, BOLD 2006 and 2007
> Organizer, Austin, Texas

I feel very passionate about birth. I think that pregnant women that see me coming duck into alleyways - not because I share my horror stories, but because I want them to study, learn, educate themselves, challenge their preconceptions - make *informed* decisions.

For my first birth, I was armed with my doula, a terrific supportive husband, my mom, and tons of knowledge. But, I wasn't prepared for the idea that opinionated me would be so inwardly focused that I would do anything to get my certified nurse midwife to just leave me alone! My son was somewhat malpositioned. No one would *let* me labor on hands and knees like I wanted. My birth got highjacked by the midwife's supervising OB and I ended up with a terrible forced c-section for my asynclitic baby (after he was crowning). My c-section was coerced and my OB was punitive (her notes indicate that if he had come down, she was going to intentionally cut a fourth degree episiotomy). My experience was terrible.

My second time around I wore the "high risk" badge of VBAC. Why are people only high or low risk, anyway? I found a wonderful homebirth midwife (CPM). I fully expected another 28 hour labor. About an hour into the labor, I was sure that I wouldn't survive if I had to do this for another 24 hours. When I was really getting overwhelmed, my husband simply whispered that he loved me, and I got grounded again. My son was born in our bathtub into my husband's hands about 30 minutes later. This was one of the most intimate experiences in our marriage.

My third birth was also a planned homebirth. I thought that he was posterior - and he was. I had a wonderful midwife and the most supportive husband in the world. No matter how much I complained that it hurt and I couldn't do it - they told me they loved me and I was doing it. I gave birth to a posterior, 10 lb. 12 oz baby at home. Now I can leap tall buildings in a single bound.

Did it hurt? Yes. But, for all of the epidurals in the world – I wouldn't trade lying in *my* bed with my new son and letting him meet his brothers or the "MY BODY ROCKS" feeling of having done it.

I love how the play reinforces that everyone's needs are different and we have to respect different people's journeys. But, at the same time, we need to give people all of the right tools to make the best choices for themselves.

I am the organizer of this play for my college's gender studies program and our local birth organization. I have three small sons and a full-time job - so, this is making me a bit overwhelmed at times. I guess I need my midwife to keep whispering in my ear - "you *are* doing it."

- Kari Benton, BOLD 2006 Organizer, Lynchburg, Virginia

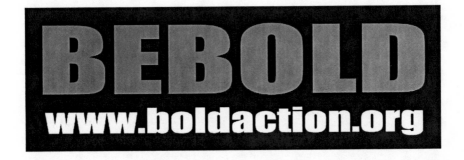

"BOLD is an exciting, uplifting, and empowering answer to the childbirth crisis. I support this movement with every fiber of my being."

- Christiane Northrup, MD, FACOG, author of *Mother-Daughter Wisdom, The Wisdom of Menopause* and *Women's Bodies, Women's Wisdom*

Join BOLD's global movement!

BOLD was born in 2006 with productions of *Birth* around the world, but today BOLD is even more than Karen Brody's play. In addition to yearly performance and talkbacks of *Birth* our initiatives include BOLD Red Tents, the BOLD College Campaign and more.

Visit our website at **www.boldaction.org** to learn how you can get involved in the BOLD movement. Add your voice and show the world the power inside your community to make childbirth the best it can be for all mothers!

ACKNOWLEDGMENTS

Every day I bow in gratitude to the many people who made it possible for me to write this play and get it out into the world. So many BOLD angels have touched me on my journey. They include: Angela Lauria, who I consider to be the co-founder of BOLD (you got me off my butt to do it!); Cate Stokes for believing in me more than I sometimes believed in myself; Melissa for our phone calls; Ruta for your loving friendship and Buddhist example; Kris for "The Partridge Family" CD you brought on our road trip to Virginia; my mother for loving everything I do; The Playwrights Forum for being there to workshop the play; Heidi Miami Marshall for your hours helping me make this script the best it can be; Kitama Jackson for filming so many BOLD events for practically nothing; Dr. Christiane Northrup for being unafraid to speak the truth about childbirth to women; Mary Alexander, Ida Darragh,

Stacey Blackburn and Jennifer in Little Rock for being with me for both of my births and showing me just how much midwifery care can rock; and all the cast and crew from every BOLD production. You all rock.

And to my family. Jacob, thank you for your generosity of spirit, loving nature and good humor. Aden, thank you for always reminding me of the importance to be present, play games and laugh. And to Tim, who puts up with my spontaneous creative pursuits, passionately believes we must have a society that honors mothers when they give birth, and never balked once at how right it was for me to dedicate my self, time and a bit of our nest egg to the play and BOLD. Thank you for your commitment to our journey, to the love you shower on me and your eagerness to do a lot of childcare and housework!

To Rose Nyaga, for always reminding me on the tough days to encourage myself. And Sister Sheila, for midwifing me through a difficult time.

There is no strength without challenges. To all my life challenges I thank you. Each and every one of them has awakened my feminine spirit.

ABOUT THE AUTHOR

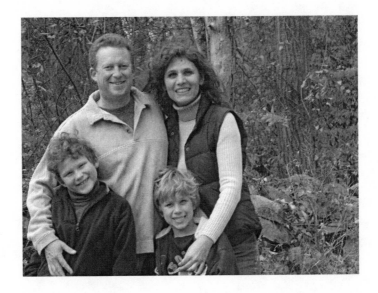

Karen Brody's critically-acclaimed play, *Birth*, is currently playing in theaters around the world as part of BOLD, a worldwide arts-based movement to improve childbirth choices and put mothers at the center of their birth experiences. She has written for Mothering Magazine and several other magazines. Brody produced a short film about BOLD, *Being BOLD*, in 2007. Before becoming a writer she was a community organizer working with women's groups in Belize, Guatemala, Kenya and New York City. Brody has a masters in Women and International Development from the Institute of Social Studies in The Netherlands. She is the founder and Artistic Director of BOLD and is currently working on a book. She lives with her husband and two children in the woods.

WEBSITES THAT ROCK

BOLD
www.boldaction.org

Mothering Magazine
www.mothering.com

White Ribbon Alliance for Safe Motherhood
www.whiteribbonalliance.org

Women Deliver
www.womendeliver.org

National Advocates for Pregnant Women (NAPW)
www.advocatesforpregnantwomen.org

Orgasmic Birth
www.orgasmicbirth.com

Childbirth Connection
www.childbirthconnection.org

International Cesarean Awareness Network
www.ican-online.org

Coalition for Improving Maternity Services
www.motherfriendly.org

The Breastfeeding Cafe
www.breastfeedingcafe.com

Solace for Mothers
www.solaceformothers.org

The Business of Being Born
www.thebusinessofbeingborn.com

Choices in Childbirth
www.choicesinchildbirth.org

Printed in the United States
121599LV00005B/37-66/P